CRYSTALS

How to Use the Power of Crystals and Healing Stones

(The Complete Guide to Becoming Conscious With Crystals)

Andrea Baker

Published by Harry Barnes

Andrea Baker

All Rights Reserved

Crystals: How to Use the Power of Crystals and Healing Stones (The Complete Guide to Becoming Conscious With Crystals)

ISBN 978-1-7751430-2-4

All rights reserved. No part of this guide may be reproduced in any form without permission in writing from the publisher except in the case of brief quotations embodied in critical articles or reviews.

Legal & Disclaimer

The information contained in this book is not designed to replace or take the place of any form of medicine or professional medical advice. The information in this book has been provided for educational and entertainment purposes only.

The information contained in this book has been compiled from sources deemed reliable, and it is accurate to the best of the Author's knowledge; however, the Author cannot guarantee its accuracy and validity and cannot be held liable for any errors or omissions. Changes are periodically made to this book. You must consult your doctor or get professional medical advice before using any of the suggested remedies, techniques, or information in this book.

Upon using the information contained in this book, you agree to hold harmless the Author from and against any damages, costs, and expenses, including any legal fees potentially resulting from the application of any of the information provided by this guide. This disclaimer applies to any damages or injury caused by the use and application, whether directly or indirectly, of any advice or information presented, whether for breach of contract, tort, negligence, personal injury, criminal intent, or under any other cause of action.

You agree to accept all risks of using the information presented inside this book. You need to consult a professional medical practitioner in order to ensure you are both able and healthy enough to participate in this program.

Table of Contents

INTRODUCTION 1

CHAPTER 1: CHOOSING YOUR CRYSTAL 4

CHAPTER 2: CRYSTAL HEALING 26

CHAPTER 3: THE POWER OF CRYSTALS 60

CHAPTER 4: HEALING GEMSTONES & CRYSTALS 77

CHAPTER 5: COLOR POWER 110

CHAPTER 6: THE HEALING POWER OF CRYSTALS DO THEY WORK? 115

CHAPTER 7: 50 CRYSTALS TO KNOW (FROM A TO Z) 132

CHAPTER 8: WHAT INFLUENCES ARE THE PLANETS ON CRYSTALS? 154

CHAPTER 9: STOP RINGING IN THE EARS - USE REMEDIES FOR TINNITUS TO STOP THE AWFUL NOISE 168

CONCLUSION 192

Introduction

The history of crystal healing is definitely a very rich and colorful one. It is astounding as to how extremely beneficial the crystal healing process can be for mankind. The concept is definitely not a new one; it dates back to the times of magicians and holy men. The most common usages of crystals in past focused on fortune telling and communication with the dead. Healing the sick is another common use of the crystal process which has been in practice for centuries now. The main reason behind its use in modern times is the protection and healing powers it offers.

Crystals have been used for over five centuries, from the ancient Egyptians to the modern man. People are more often than not aware of the phenomenon of crystal healing on a very basic level, but it is something worth taking a deeper look into and exploring for yourself.

With the immensely vast collection of crystals available, it becomes rather difficult for a person with limited knowledge to choose the ideal option for his or her particular need. There are certain crystals known for establishing the foundation of the healing and protection process. Then there are others known for additional properties that are specific to a type of healing or protection. A library could be easily filled purely on the subject of crystals. There are innumerable suppliers and vendors of crystals, and a specified set of crystals that are particularly to fit the demands of a beginner.

Novice crystal users lack the solid understanding of crystal healing necessary to ensure optimal benefits. However, with the usage of appropriate crystals, beginners can tap into the amazing healing energies of these majestic stones. Not all stones offer the same kind of energies, and this variance makes them easy to use.

It is unnecessary to search the internet aimlessly looking for accurate information. This guide provides readers with all of the essential information about, and a thorough understanding of the right approach to, crystals and their properties..

After exploring different crystals and their meanings and functionality, you can easily master crystal healing at the beginner level. You can also determine the perfect crystal for your life and needs, discover the optimal ways to activate and charge your special stone, manage and enhance the value of the precious stones for profit, become acquainted with methods using the crystals to perform tasks, and learn how to clean and maintain the crystals in order to preserve their powers.

Chapter 1: Choosing Your Crystal

Choosing the proper crystal(s) is as important as choosing the correct tools for a job. You can't hammer a nail with a wood saw and working with crystals is no different. Using the wrong crystals at the wrong time may not only impair the likelihood of achieving our goals but could also stop any progress dead in its tracks. However, when chosen effectively crystals can and often do supercharge numerous aspects of life. Choosing a crystal is like choosing an extension of one's self and should be looked at as a type of ceremony. It should only be done in a peaceful atmosphere preferably with some privacy. The key to actually choosing a crystal(s) is a balance of sensory acuity and intuition. We must listen to our feelings as not all crystals suit all moods when in the wrong mood some crystals can bring on feelings ranging from lethargy to mood swings and depression. Below is a step by step guide designed to simplify the process of choosing the correct crystals, crystals that resonate with our individual wishes and goals in order to enable us to manifest and maintain our desires by boosting our natural (and in some cases innate) ability to transform and shape our reality and the lives of our loved ones. The first thing to do is cleanse and charge all of your crystals and lay them out, either on the floor or on a sizable cloth, then proceed.

Before choosing a crystal, we must first emotionally balance ourselves and take a few minutes to practice breathing exercises and meditation. This will calm the thought process and help to provide the clarity needed for the next step.

Whilst in meditation begin to focus your energy on your desired outcome, intent or desire. This will affect your overall energetic frequency and vibrational state by bringing it closer to that of your previously stated outcome, intent and desires.

When you feel comfortable and have achieved the desired mood and frame of mind, turn to your crystals, put your hands together in the prayer position and request guidance from the crystals themselves in choosing the best-suited crystal or a mix of crystals for carrying out your wishes.

Gently close your eyes and using your non-dominant hand (palm facing down) and slowly move it over the stones until you feel a pull from a crystal. The pull is generated by the crysta'ls vibrational energy harmonising with the vibrational field of the body, which is why it is so important to properly centre ourselves before choosing crystals. The more in tune our emotions and energetic field are with our desired outcomes and goals the better as this creates clearer more defined connections between our energetic selves and our crystals. You might pick just one crystal or you may pick 2, 3 or more, you will know when you have chosen enough and when it feels like time to move on to the next stage.

If you are having difficulty in feeling the 'pull' of a crystal, try picking up each stone one at a time and hold it in your hand taking notice of the feelings and effects it induces.

Once you have chosen a number of crystals lay them out in front of you and repeat the steps above again but his time when moving your hand over the stones and feel which of the stones gives the greatest pull be aware that some crystals may have a pull that feels more like a tingling sensation rather than an actual pull, however, in most case (as with myself) generally a light pull is felt much in the same way as a dousing rod directs skilled users towards water and oil.

Take notice of which stones have the greatest connection and pull to your current mindset and desires and separate them from the rest. Return the leftover crystals to their usual storage box, bag, etc.

Another option is to experiment, however, this haphazard will no doubt prove be time-consuming and produce hit and miss results at the best of times. A more efficient option would be to do a little research on your crystals in order to properly ascertain which crystals are best suited to your particular task. Luckily, the last section of this book is comprised of a comprehensive crystal guide packed full of vital information and was written with the beginner in mind but is also in-depth enough to enlighten even the most experienced of practitioners.

Actinolite

This is a crystal that displays numerous shades of green but can also appear in black, white, grey, brown or blue and forms in needle-like clusters branching out in all directions. Sometimes known as Tremolite, Actinolite acts as a powerful psychic shield which brings balance to our actions by boosting decision making and strategic skills. Those who meditate with Actinolite can expect to feel surges of positive feelings which can often leave to experiencing the higher planes of spiritual awareness. Actinolite not only brings with it feelings of positivity but also has the ability to relieve those suffering from stress or 'emotional burnout'. It is believed that Actinolite stimulates the body's natural detoxification process, cleanses the liver, kidneys, and works great for energy restoration. Actinolite has the ability to break destructive patterns and behaviours and is also a seeker crystal which helps to guide us towards fortuitous situations and positive change. Emotionally Actinolite soothes tempers and brings an air of dependability which creates stability making Actinolite an excellent choice for those suffering from addictions, grief, and guilt. Actinolite is closely linked to the Throat Chakra which, when activated and balanced brings the rest of the chakras into alignment and allows for the free flow of energy throughout the body. The connection to the Throat Chakra also stimulates truth both within us and in our relationships with others.

Colour

Shades of Green

Black

Blue

Brown

Grey

White

Zodiac

Scorpio

Energetic Frequencies

Protective

Balance

Calming

Chakra

The Heart Chakra

The Throat Chakra

Adamite

Adamite is a stone revered for its effect on creativity and left brain thinking. It is a highly popular gem for many reasons as it has powerful effects on us emotionally, spiritually and psychically but also for its fluorescent qualities. Under UV (Ultra Violet) light Adamite displays incandescent hues and magical light refractions. Typically a green stone, Adamite also forms in blue (rare) violet, pink and yellow. Adamite holds strong connections to the emotions to and has a powerful influence over the emotions of those that are lucky enough to come in contact with it. It stimulates creativity and clarity of thought and strengthens determination making

Adamite the perfect stone for those facing a stressful or difficult situation or individuals. Primarily Adamite activates the Solar Plexus Chakra but is also linked to the Heart and Throat Chakra, promoting truth and loyalty through our thoughts and actions. It helps us to not overact in the heat of the moment and also pushes us to seek out new challenges and experiences. Adamite's vibrational energy envelops the wearer in feelings of safety and serenity as it dispels feelings of depression, excessive guilt and irrational fear. It is a powerful protective stone that works well as a meditative aid and is said to bring on lucid dreams if a stone is left by the bedside. Adamite's connection to the Heart Chakra allows it to exert beneficial effects, stabilising heart rate and reducing blood pressure. The energy radiating from Adamite acts as a balance on both the emotional system and the body network as a whole. It soothes throat conditions, laryngitis, and thyroid related illnesses as well as chest infections and is also thought to be useful to those suffering from persistent headaches. It is the perfect stone for those embarking on a new adventure or starting a new business.

Colour

Green

Blue

Pink

Violet

Yellow

White/Colourless

Zodiac

Cancer

Energetic Frequencies

Healing

Protection

Affluence

Chakras

The Throat Chakra

The Solar Plexus Chakra

The Heart Chakra

Aegirine

This stunningly elegant gemstone is black to dark green in colour and is known to possess extremely strong protective energies. By guarding the wearer's chakra network, aura, and physical body in times of danger and difficulty Aegirine has earnt its reputation of instilling confidence, conviction and courage in those affected by its cool, light-hearted energy. Usually found in Canada, Greenland, Russia, Scotland, and Nigeria, Aegirine as a name is derived from the Norse sea god Aegir and has also been called Acmite after the Greek word meaning 'point' which is an apt description as Aegirine is commonly found sticking out of rock, looking not unlike blades protruding from the earth itself. Aegirine is a great crystal for overcoming self-consciousness and the unnecessary shame that comes from facing the overzealous judgements of others of our appearance and/or lifestyle choices.

Aegirine has been used in the treatment of immune deficiencies, as protection against psychic attacks covering jealousy, malicious intent and all manner of curses, and is well known for its ability to combine and magnify the healing properties of other gemstones when numerous healing stones are used together. Other attributes of Aegirine include the ability to purge any pessimistic attachments and feelings of disappointment whilst simultaneously acting as a shield against electrical sensitivity caused by the 'electromagnetic soup' (radiation from electronics, wi-fi and cell phone signals) in which we all live. Wearing Aegirine will boost your feelings of wellbeing and joy which makes it an ideal talisman for those suffering from stress or addiction.

Colour

Black

Dark Green

Birthstone

No association

Zodiac

Pisces

Energetic frequencies

Power

Protection

Truth

Healing

Chakra

The Base or Root Chakra

Agate

Agate is a name commonly used to cover many different varieties of Chalcedony which display an almost endless array of colours, pure, banded, mixed or colourless. Sometimes called the 'earth rainbow' it is said that Agate and its vast colour spectrum is the gemstone embodiment of the varying states of our innermost world. Agate possesses a lower vibrational frequency than most gemstones, however, its energy is extremely influential in balancing the aura, has a stabilising effect which promotes responsibility, reliability, maturity, and also acts as an amazing conduit for spiritual energies which leads to thoughts of self-encouragement and feelings of self-confidence. The supporting energy of Agate is perfect for pregnancy and for new mums, it stimulates lactation, and helps to combat stress such as the 'baby blues'. Agate adds clarity to mental processes, boosting memory, decision-making skills and logic making it especially helpful in gathering one's thoughts before important meetings. There are hundreds of different types of Agate with many having their own unique properties, however, Agate, in general, is said to repel insects, ease stomach illnesses, cure skin problems, and can reduce fever. As mentioned above there are hundreds if not thousands of types of Agate, below is just a few of the better-known examples.

Blue Agate

Blue Agate or 'Blue Lace' displays light, subtle hues of exquisite sky blue that carries within it calming energies which support and encourage the user and it is said that wearing Blue Agate can make one more articulate. Through its synchronicity with the Throat Chakra Blue Agate is able to soothe sore throats and swollen glands, reduce symptoms relating to arthritis, and lessen or eliminate frequent headaches and migraines. Blue Agate can also have a positive effect on an individual's emotional wellbeing by opening the Brow Chakra and can bring peace to an overactive imagination in times of worry.

Crazy Lace Agate

Crazy Lace Agate is a wonderful stone overflowing with joyous energy earning it the name of 'Laughter stone' and in some circles even 'Happy Lace'. It is packed with twists and turns of varying colours sometimes predominantly white, at times more reddish or brown or grey to black and on occasion hues of gold and yellow. Crazy Lace Agate activates both the Crown and Third Eye Chakra the energies of which combine to elevate the mind with an interest towards unification, collaboration, laughter, and a hunger for variety. Negative vibrational energy dissipates in the presence of Crazy Lace Agate as its calming yet joyous vibrations inspire composure and communication. When carried or worn as a talisman Crazy Lace Agate combats sudden scares and helps one in overcoming phobias and irrational fears.

Laguna Agate

Laguna Agate is renowned for its narrow and compact bands consisting of vivid shades of cardinal reds and crimson. Wearing Laguna Agate is thought to boost blood flow and stamina leaving the wearer feeling revitalised. It is also believed to provide protection for travellers. Laguna Agate's energetic frequency opens and activates the Base Chakra clearing any emotional blockages and has a stabilising effect on the body's energetic network and aura, ridding one of any feelings of unworthiness and discontent.

Colour

Clear

Sky Blue

Red

Brown

Orange

Green

Black

Grey

Gold

Yellow

Multi-coloured

Zodiac

Gemini

Birthstone

February (Blue 'Lace' Agate)

March (Blue 'Lace' Agate)

September (Laguna Agate)

October (Laguna Agate)

November (Laguna Agate)

Energetic Frequencies

Supportive

Love

Healing

Encouragement

Chakras

General association with all the chakras through its effect on the aura as a whole.

The Crown Chakra (Crazy Lace Agate)

The Brow or Third Eye Chakra (Blue 'Lace' Agate, Crazy Lace Agate)

The Throat Chakra (Blue 'Lace' Agate)

The Root or Base Chakra (Laguna Agate)

Albite

Albite is a type of Feldspar that forms in an array of colours including colourless, white, blue, grey, pink, and a mixture of red and browns. When Albite was first discovered the white version of the gemstone was most common, however since then many other colours have been found, the varying colourings being due to inclusions and imperfections within the crystal itself. Albite activates the Crown Chakra, stimulating brain activity, because of this, it is said that Albite enhances all manner of mental attributes, boosting memory and promoting clear-headedness as well as supporting concise, logical thinking. Further to the effects already mentioned above Albite when meditated with acts as a powerful conduit to the higher spiritual realms. Keeping Albite by your bedside eliminates insomnia and encourages lucid dreaming. Albite is regularly used in psychic readings, astral projections, past life regressions, remote viewing, and all manner of spiritual healing treatments and rituals. Albites connections to the brain pass over into the physical realm. It is believed to speed up the recovery from head and brain injuries as well as being extremely useful to those suffering from mental illness and/or trauma. As a crystal that brings people together, the energy emitted by Albite creates an air of cooperation for the greater good, selflessness, team building, comradery, and family ties. What a wonderful thing to behold! Albite has also been used in the treatment of eye conditions as well as to promote blood detoxification and aid in healing brain damage. It has a positive effect on almost all of the body's natural process from stimulating metabolism and balancing stomach acids to strengthening the apatite and is even thought to help those suffering from Alzheimer's and other degenerative illnesses relating to the brain.

Colour

Colourless

White

Blue

Grey

Pink

Red/Brown

Zodiac

Aquarius

Birthstone

January

February

Energetic Frequencies

Healing

Spiritual

Chakras

The Crown Chakra

Chapter 2: Crystal Healing

The concept of Kristal Healing has made it onto the area of irrational superstition and "the new age hooey" for many of us who have spent their lives on the physical plane we like to call "reality." It is as if most of us are asking how in the universe a stone can be much less power than a rock and allow us to heal. How can stones, minerals, and metals, except sit down?

To respond to this issue, we should go beyond the physical existence in which we conclude that "all is" in this world in which we reside.

The physical matter has long been recognized as a stable foundation of nature. In other words, physicality is the measure most of us use to distinguish "real" from "not real." Yet the material matter is not, as we know, the center of reality. Rather, it is just a small aspect of infinite energy in the universe. Material existence could be thought of like the ultra-thin membrane of this world, much like hair. The epidermis surface that covers the intangible substructure of other massive dimensions where energy vibrates differently, depending on the dimensions. Every physical object, whether living or not, does not only exist at this physical level but also in the many energetic dimensions beyond physicality. Everything you see is multidimensional in this universe. Your entire body system is nothing but energy that occurs in different patterns and densities. The same applies to what we see as "inanimate objects" as stones.

We experience what we call wellbeing when patterns of energy work together in a non-resistant and coherent way. Such energy cycles can be disrupted by many issues. In this situation, we are in a state of discomfort. It results in poor nutrition. This sensitive, discordant energy pattern is responsible for any negative symptoms that we encounter from headaches to cancer in our bodies.

What we believe to be true simply appears for us, our physical senses do nothing but see energy as a scent or a sight or taste our physical senses. It is our senses which turn what is an energetic holographic reality for lack of better words into the static reality that we call material. The senses tell us that we are "separate" from the world. We are not only interested in this large energy field at our most important level, but also this energetic field. Each animated and inanimate object we see is one of us. Our physical lives are only different expressions of the same force that comprises "all that is" in every universe and dimension. The magnitude and frequency of this energy (what we often call vibration) are what decides whether energy becomes an individual or stone in physical dimensions.

Crystals are free of resistant patterns and what they call gemstones. They are among the most stable, coherent, solid and deliberate systems in the physical dimension. The changeless physical structure reflects the fact that its inherent energetic patterns of balance, power, and cohesion are incorruptible. In the physical dimension, it may seem like you're only really handling a different, physical object when you take up a crystal. In the other dimensions, though, where both you and the rock live, you "practice" with this rock vigorously. This practice then affects the physical aspect of structure and psychology. The law governing all facets of the universe is that of "unity." We have come to call it the "Rule of Attraction" in physical life. Simply put, only vibrational frequencies can coexist. To share the same space with another "shape," you must, therefore, vibrate on the same level as you vibrate. Health is the natural condition of every form in the universe. The natural inclination and purpose for anything within the universe is, therefore, harmony, cohesiveness, and capability. This ensures that the natural development of the vibration is stimulated and resonated against wellbeing. Therefore, when you divide the space into a crystal (or gemstone), which has a resistance-free vibration, the energy will absorb and take its cohesive pattern, instead of vibration of the crystal that adopts a non-cohesive pattern. Such practice allows you not to establish a pain pattern within your energy substructures any longer and thus the physical manifestation of this unrelieved energy is no longer sustained, and the physical symptom disappears. Thanks to this effect, crystals and gemstones are incredibly well-adapted to bring us back into vibratory health and harmony. Anything that has a non-resistance energy pattern will act as a tuning fork, providing of the vibration that can be used to adapt to a healthy vibration. This is what happens when you hear a song that makes you feel good and spend time next to a person who makes yourself feel good or taking a homeopathic remedy.

Each crystal or gemstone resonates energetically in a slightly different fashion, so it is different from the physical in terms of things like chemistry, geometry, structure, light, and fabric (just like our specific physical structures). That is why everyone gives themselves to patterns that exist in our physical structures. For example, sharing the room with rose quartz means revealing the energetic patterns in our physical and metaphorical core to comply with the health and follow a resistance freestyle. Therefore, unresolved heart problems will dissipate if equipped with a pink half, allowing us to let go of whatever distorts our energies that associate with the heart.

Crystals and gemstones develop deep in the earth's crust at extremely high pressures and heat over millions of years. This gives them a position with the most intrinsic energy among earthly objects. We can receive, produce, project, emanate, refract and reflect heat. Crystals have a highly consistent atomic structure. In the gemstone, which is known as "quartz," these atoms vibrate at a steady and observable frequency, making quartz an ideal recipient and emitter of electromagnetic energy. Therefore, quartz is used in clocks, watches and many other technologies. Nobel laureate physicist Marcel Vogel discovered that it is not only possible to program crystals as silicon chips on computers, but also that the power of consciousness can be programmed. He discovered that if a person uses a computer, thought by pressing the keyboard is sent to the machine. Then Vogel correctly argued that, like electricity, thought can be driven by what we call energy. According to this observation, he concluded that crystals could be programmed, using only thoughts as information power, without the need for electricity.

Quartz is a piezoelectric material. A piezoelectric material generates an electrical charge when it is met with mechanical stress. If the piezoelectric material is put under mechanical stress, the positive and negative charging centers in the material change and an internal electric field result. This strain can be caused by the material being bent and rotated to bend the crystal structure without breaking it. The mechanism also acts oppositely, when a small electric current is applied, with the product deforming slightly. While the point is that the piezoelectric effect plays or does not play a role in a human-crystal healing relationship, there are significant consequences that crystals respond so well to electromagnetic fields. This has serious repercussions because our bodies consist of electro-magnetic fields, crystals and gemstones, and they constantly emanate, react to this power that creates and runs through our bodies. Another interesting finding is the fact that quartz consists of silicon and oxygen (SiO_2, which are the building block of all minerals known to geologists. Our world consists of silicon and oxygen-containing minerals. Silicon is a major component of our human bodies. Several researchers have theorized that the transfer of energy within our bodies from natural crystal to silicone can have something to do with the physical healing effect that crystal exposure can have.

Crystals and gemstones are among the strongest physical tools available to us. It is a device that we all used unintentionally at some point. It is often an interaction that takes place by drawing our attention to a certain object. We think it's "cool" on the physical level, and although we don't know why it so much we want, we feel obliged to pick it up and hold it in our pocket. We don't know why we felt the impulse, and we don't know what is behind our drive to take it. We have no idea that our energy substructure invites us to the vibration of this rock to shift with it into a better and coherent pattern than the one we hold in ourselves. Like all tools, the secret to optimizing use is to learn how to apply the device consciously. If this scenario could go beyond an involuntary desire to a conscious process of searching for a certain crystal or gemstone based upon awareness of its use, the receptivity of the individual would become a hundredfold. Once we learn that the energy-grade for each crystal and gemstone influences its electromagnetic fields, we would see that we produce a techno-chemical effect inside our body and psychology that will allow us to use it as the powerful tools they are. We can use them every day to promote health, knowledge, growth, and development within ourselves and in our multi-dimensional lives.

Emery Boards Vs Metal Files Vs Crystal Nail Files

You can own a crystal nail file yourself or have a trial spin at a women's show or a regional fair. It's elegant, colorful and very trendy, but worth $7 and is superior to thousands of emery panels that we buy?

Emery boards are cartons with small sand grains stuck to them, and they are practically compatible with sandpaper. When you file, the nail breaks the emery board, that is how it files.

You need to file in one direction with emery boards to prevent nail damage during filing. Sandpaper on a stick called an emery board comes in different grate so that you can file your nail down in size, form it, and do your best to tame the sharp, jagged edges that you always use with an emery board.

Emery boards are rough on your hands, but the work is done. The roughness of your file depends also on whether you have soft, thin, delicate nails or smooth, sturdy hooves.

Unfortunately, they are designed to do emery boards, which damage your nails more than anything. If you use an emery board, you leave the nail tip "open" rather than "locked," just as pores are open and shut on the body. Leaving the edge of the nail "open" ensures that inside the nail dirt and water will leak itself causing the nails to spray, crack and peel and weaken. The harshness of the sandpaper's grinding motion weakens the tooth.

Due to the porous nature of the carton, glue, and dust, dirt and debris can be mixed into the file and mushrooms and bacteria can grow rapidly. Although you might not see it with your eyes, a good microbiologist and a microscope will illuminate you on a street! There is no way to clean up the emery board, let alone sanitize it, and they are so bacteria that after every use you must throw out the emery board. This is the standard procedure in professional salons by the FDA and it takes us to the environmental factor. On the "green-o-meter," the emery board is very small. The number of trees used to make millions of files and the landfill space occupied by the tiny 5-inch sticks is larger than you can imagine.

Metal files on a stick mate, the emery plate, slightly better than their bacteria.

The metal files are manufactured in two ways: one is made from small flakes of metal attached to a metal or cardboard stick, two is created with a metal stick and the stick is rugged to create a filing area. In both cases, little, tiny bits of metal flake off while filing. Glass, although it is much stronger and more resilient than sand granules, is typical of a lower degree and is still very fragile as far as glass is concerned.

Metal files often grind the nail and leave the tip of the nail "open" rather than "closed." Because of the metal bits on the record, dust and debris can be stuck between the tiny "teeth" like iron and can stick to the sheet. Metal is non-porous, so bacteria can't grow on the file itself but bacteria can grow on nail waste and any dirt trapped in the folder. You can rinse out a metal folder, but you must be careful not to develop rust in any cracks between the "teeth."

The metal files can not be cleanly sanitized to the satisfaction of the FDA.

On green metal records, the number of trees that are used in their development was slightly higher than their cardboard relative. Aluminum does some nasty chemicals during the manufacturing process, and aluminum files should be discarded after several applications because they can not be sanitized efficiently. It takes a lot longer for them to decompose in places than emery boards.

The crystal files are cut off from the actual crystal and the surface of the crystal is handled to roughen the filing layer during processing.

The crystal nail file glides over the tip of the finger. It doesn't break the nail like the emery board or metal pad, so you can file in both ways and as a bonus. You will note how smooth the nail tips are when you file your nails with the crystal file. The crystal file covers the tip of the nail and screens it, stopping moisture and dirt from escaping into your claw.

Crystal is very hygienic and non-porous. No bacteria or debris may grow on the surface of the filing or become stuck on the crystal file rough layer. The same applies to the crystal pumice file that may be left in the bathroom without any fear of mold, mildew, fungus or bacteria being grown there or there!

Your crystal nail files are made of recycled quartz. Some factories make them from fresh, large sheets of glass, but after making vases and stub ware, the highest quality crystal factories have found an application for the remaining crystal. The crystal is melted into large sheets. The different sizes of nail files and pumice files were taken from these plates.

There are no different crystal data samples, except the pumice file.

Crystal nail files comply with all FDA sanitation requirements. They can be sanitized in ethanol, baked in an autoclave under UV light. Due to their hygienic nature, crystal files, especially the pumice file, are ideal for diabetics. You don't have to think about yourself slicing, as diabetics do while caring for your feet.

If not a lifetime, crystal nail files will last years. Crystal is very difficult when finding in nature. Once the crystal is formed in the earth, the cooling rate is slower so that the crystal molecules have more time to form tight, solid-bonded lattice structures. Crystal is the superior material compared to glass, which cools very quickly and the molecules have no time to make up the robust support system for gills.

The crystal nail file has high grades of green-o-meter due to the use of plumbing free, environmentally safe teeth in its made from recycled materials and several plants. We last so long that waste disposal is not greatly affected by excessive use, such as your friends on cardboard or metal pin. A crystal nail and pumice file could last the life of a person!

Crystal-Healing the Chakras

According to old texts, the chakras appear as spinning light wheels. The word chakra is simply Sanskrit for the rim. Chakras obtain and emit energy that, depending on the quality of this power, maybe either negative or positive. You will discover variations in each chakra's needs during the healing process. You don't have to be afraid of this challenge. Think of your chakras as a garden with every flower that needs special care. Many chakras need less focus, others are more demanding. The devotion to this self-examination makes the chakras so challenging as to be satisfying.

The following instructions can be changed to suit your needs. When picking stones, be careful not about their size or appearance, but your reaction when keeping them. Some of these crystals may not be common, but they can probably be found in a mystical or rock store. Whilst you can appreciate this guide to chakra healing, a trained professional is ideally able to undertake a long-term procedure. Most skilled chakra healers are highly intuitive as well as experienced. Your analytical perspective will help you understand why each disparity exists. It can be soothing in itself.

Chakra 1st: This is the chakra heart. It's at the base of your backbone and tailbone. This chakra needs little attention when you feel grounded, protected and embedded at the moment. But many aren't so lucky. A blocked root chakra can make you understand the real, cling and overly possessive. Conversely, if you're too free, your body and belongings may be alienated. As a consequence, your kindness can be used.

Crystal Correction: Obsidian opens a blocked chakra. This gem offers a focused, calm outlook so that an appreciation of the fleeting nature of things removes the desire to gain compellingly. Place obsidian on the genital area to remove blocks when listing on your back. When you relax the power of the stone interacts with your own, it is strengthened. Rose quartz is required for an abundantly open core. This delicate, pink quartz, while usually linked to the brain, helps us to accept and love ourselves so we can defend ourselves by saying no. 2 Chakra: The sacral chakra governs our sexual energy and creativeness. You just have to press two inches under your navel to know where it is. The gift of a healthy sacred chakra is elegance and language. A blockage may lead to resistance to new ideas. A sacred chakra which exposed is evident from bed-hopping to dangerous driving in the "drama queen," as well as in any risky behavior.

Crystal Correction: Carnelian: this quartz variety is lovely for opening the sacred region. Although it can be found in many colors, red or orange stimulating qualities offer shy courage. This helps us to pursue our dreams without the delusions that obstruct our direction. On the other hand, if this chakra is too open, lapis Luigi may be needed. In ancient Egypt and Babylon, this legendary light-blue rock was highly prized. Today, we can use their moderating powers to help us behave carefully. "Taking this stone to the body simply improves the cognitive, physical, spiritual, psychological and emotional conditions."

3rd Chakra: This is your solar plexus, also referred to as the center of power. A pool of untapped will and bravery remains here. We know our potential and are inspired to fulfill it when this chakra is safe. If we are trapped we can feel "butterflies in our belly" or another stomach distresses. A blocked power center makes us feel weak and helpless. The opposite is when this energy center is too big.

Golden Beryl is a sweet, lemon yellow stone that guides and enhances confidence. It is good for 3rd chakra blockages, therefore. Place this two-inch-high stone above your navel will free your energy center to help you achieve your objectives. Green jade is for those confused by this chakra. A calming stone can quickly and harmlessly channel our emotions and growing harmful feelings towards others.

4th Chakra: this is the chakra of the heart and its location. This is the sacred domain of spiritual development, devotion, strength and high ideals. A stormy core chakra enables us and us highly dangerous. In this case, it is hard for us to open up spaces for love and friendship. On the other hand, when our heart is too big, we can try to carry the weight of the world and do the impossible.

Crystal Correction: Green jasper put on the heart allows us to feel safe and show ourselves. It makes frank and enjoyable contact simpler. Seek peridot for a heart without limits. The soft, pastel green stone always calms us down. Peridot helps us to be nice but not sacrificial.

5th Chakra: the chakra of the throat allows us to connect through both word and speech. It's at the bottom of the throat. We speak honestly and freely when this chakra is healthy. The deception is subtle if we are blocked here. For example, we can leave details out. Instead, we talk too much if this chakra is bloated and without excitement. This is often referred to as' foot in the ear ' syndrome.

Crystal Correction: a magnificent navy rock, sodalite, helps with a wide throat chakra. This crystal provides us with confidence and clarity. We can sound it with certainty, knowing our reality. Those with a broad 5th chakra should, on the other hand, sound their truth quieter. Amber is helpful in this capacity. This stone is very soulful.

6th Chakra: This power core is regarded to many as the third eye between the brows. If this chakra is aligned, it allows us to see past appearances and exposes our inherent spiritual ability. However, if it is blocked, we restrict ourselves to evidence that is not investigated. It leads to linear thinking and happiness. If we are too accessible here, though, we might be isolated from the physical world. The inability to close the psychic eye floods with a disturbing sense of unreality when necessary. Balance is key. Balance is key. We also have to wake Crystal Correction, as we dream: moonlight on the sixth chakra will clear the problems that blind our intuition and unseen the spirit.

Because moonstone is linked to changing cycles, it invites personal growth. It allows us to adapt to motion, spontaneity, and rigidity. Blue lace agate is appropriate with an overly open 3rd eye. The beautiful blue sky rock sharpens our attention and removes the fog of intangible interference.

Chakra 7: Oh! Wow! Words are not adequate to convey the chakra's strength. This chakra is located at the top of your head and offers the possibility of illumination. Even if it doesn't make us a Buddha, it will surely take us to heights of spiritual bliss and bind us with the meaning of our lives. You're far from alone if you're stuck here. A safe chakra of the crown is unusual. It is a blessing of unfailing efforts in the creation of the soul. When we are trapped, our life can be distorted and there is no permanent, rapturous calm. We must first ensure the well-being of our previous chakras to achieve maximum results in the balance of this chakra. It's rarely a problem to have this chakra too open if you hate happiness and harmony. Nevertheless, they live among the disillusioned. We need both the cynic and the sorrowful to communicate. If not, we will be stuck in our heads. As safe as this is, it can be quite lonely.

Crystal Correction: Clear quartz is a good healer for all chakras but it is especially useful when the closed crown is opened. The chosen crystal should be small enough to sit on the top of your head because of the 7th chakra. The stone clarifies the intent and helps us to see the wider meaning of everyday events. It helps us to learn and live in harmony with universal truths. Healing is hepatitis for those with the excessively open crown chakra. It's grounding, too. The dark and strong stone will allow us to fulfill our own and otherworldly needs, drawing attention to the practical realities of life.

Benefits of Crystals and Stones

Agate-This crystals will activate your faith, stimulate your internal talents, unleash your imagination and encourage you to think and evaluate more effectively. In addition to alleviating stresses and worries, Agate will allow you to succeed in all respects.

Amber-This mighty crystal takes up all negativity around you and replaces it with positivity-these forces allow the body to heal itself. Amber is also a very strong Feng Shui treatment for your anxiety for those who have suicidal feelings.

Amethyst — This stone will make your mind clearer and your attitude calmer, so your imagination and your information will run. It is an ideal Feng Shui therapy for those suffering from insomnia and frequent hallucinations because it will promote peace and peace of mind.

Aquamarine — The benefits of this crystal will benefit those who have difficulty expressing their feelings and speaking loudly. You will develop self-confidence and perseverance by repressing their anxieties and calming them. Aquamarine is a good time to use during experiments and meditation.

Aventurine-This crystal is very useful for focus and concentration, enabling quick decision-making and increased creativity flow. Therefore, your ability to lead others will be strengthened, and you will be able to overcome obstacles.

Bloodstone-In addition to being an excellent blood cleanser, this magic stone has the power to protect you from evil spirits and to suppress malicious thoughts.

Carnelian—This stone can promote perseverance, confidence, imagination, and leadership for those searching for the resources for advancing life so that you can better evaluate and appreciate the circumstances in your world.

Charoite—This rock is an effective Feng Shui cure for those who experience obsessive acts and compulsions. It also represses pressure by increasing any negative energy in your life and revitalizing your chi. Used Charoite leaves you happy and restless.

Clear Quartz-This lovely crystal has a strong force that can in many ways transform heat. It will also shield you from those who want to hurt you and cause you sorrow.

Garnet-This stone is a symbol of love, passion, and well-being. This removes any depression and stress in your life and increases your feelings of desire, attraction, and intimacy, helping you to feel closer and happier.

Hematite-This crystal, owing to its capacity to rejuvenate body oxygen and improve circulation, is highly regarded as a physical healer, by stimulating the absorption of iron by red blood cells.

Jade-This stone has been long wanted in ancient China for its ability to heal and protect. This pillar, a symbol of the beautiful and pure soul, will also provide mental clarity and a stronger flow of intelligence and creativity.

Jasper-This stone is a good cure for those suffering from headaches, migraines, and anxiety, it will relax their minds and promote relaxation, helping them to release their anxieties and feel more at peace with their souls.

Lapis Lazuli-This crystal symbolizes a strong spirit, as it strengthens your sense of adventure and helps you to feel more relaxed about your own life. Therefore, your fears will be diminished and you will see the world more clearly.

Moonstone-This branch, most often used as a Feng Shui treatment for women, addresses many of the issues they face: time cramps, menopause tension, and fertility barriers. Therefore, females who are using the Moonstone enhance their feminine qualities, activate internal instinct and become more physically attractive.

Obsidian-This stone is the perfect Feng Shui therapy for those who have low self-esteem and need improved confidence. Therefore, it's the perfect protection against negative chi in your life and defends you from people with evil intentions.

Onyx—The Onyx stone is a great Feng Shui cure for those who have recently got out of difficult relationships and are trying to move on. It will also maintain negative energy and keep the outlook optimistic and happy.

Peridot — This stone is commonly used by those who want to transcend the past, to let go of revolts and ancient feelings. Your heart will be free, clean, and no anger, envy, or wrath will be new.

Prehnite-This stone will ensure you are prepared for any scenario. It is also called the "unconditional love" rock and can heal any injuries and emotional problems. Therefore, Prehnite will increase your intuition.

Rhodochrosite-this stone, in Feng Shui, is a symbol of love and romanticism and continuous intercourse. It is also used to boost self-esteem and psychological needs for people who suffer from depression or denial following tragic events.

Rose Quartz-known as the' Love Stone,' this lovely product helps people with all kinds of romanticism, helps people pursue their partner in life, increases their long-term relationship value and fixes broken hearts.

Ruby-A crystal that revitalizes life, this brand brings joy to those who are searching for a greater purpose and fulfillment in their undertakings. It will help you to achieve your goals and ambitions and protect your assets against robbery or loss.

Rutilated Quartz: This stone has properties that substitute optimistic and romantic feelings with sadness, insomnia, remorse, and sad feelings. As a result, Quartz Rutilated has the potential to rekindle friendships and create a new sense of hope and imagination.

Saphire-This crystal, which is known as the "rock of wisdom," induces just that; a sense of mental clarity that removes all negatives and gives you a new mentality. Although Sapphire usually reduces mental stress, Sapphire blue is known to intensify the love emotions.

Smoky Quartz — This crystal is a good remedy for those who are lazily and lethargically impaired. By removing electromagnetic smog, an electromagnetic field that has dangerous effects on some, it creates a more focused and common-sense environment.

Sodalite-This stone helps people to discover and communicate their inner truths and stand by them regardless of circumstance. It is also a useful pillar for removing all electromagnetic fields, especially those generated by technology.

Tiger's Eye-Those who use the Tiger's Eye experience a new life drive and seek success. Through strengthening your faith, commitment, determination, and positivity, you will take your passion and make it happen.

Turkish-Many uses this lovely crystal to revitalize their chi and to create a sense of harmony. Turkey is also a cure for broken ties, building trust and hope. Use this stone to better communicate with your people.

Watermelon Tourmaline—Using this stone will help you to cope with compassion and flexibility for those who want to find new loves and embrace a relationship. You will also love yourself more and feel more joy and peace.

Zoisite—This crystal is an effective remedy for those with lethargy and depression; it reduces anxiety and encourages constructive energy. Therefore, you can achieve greater focus and imagination by using Zoisite.

Chapter 3: The Power Of Crystals

Crystals have always had incredible power and have been used as aids in healing and for rituals by hundreds of cultures all around the world. There are many who believe that this power is nothing more than superstitious nonsense, but the fact that the art of crystal healing has spread so far and lasted so long is proof that there is some truth behind the superstition

What Is Crystal Healing?

Crystal healing means to use the unique abilities of different crystals to restore, align, and transform the mind, body, and spirit, as well as to alter or improve natural energy. There are many different ways in which crystals can help you heal and improve your life, and there are hundreds of different crystals to do different things, so much so that you can fill a whole library with all the available knowledge on the subjects. To use healing crystals most effectively, it is best to receive proper training or receive the help of someone who has been properly trained and who has had ample experience using healing crystals. Don't worry, though, because even if you have no training or experience in crystal healing, there are still a lot of things you can do to use crystals to heal and improve yourself and your life. Crystals can also be a very effective first aid tool in emergency situations.

How Does Crystal Healing Work?

Although crystal healing looks, feels, and acts like magic, there is an explanation of how it works. The keywords here are energy, vibration, and resonance. It may not look like it, but everything in this world is made up of energy, including people and crystals. The atoms that form the building blocks of everything vibrate at different frequencies, producing a certain type of energy. The energy within a crystal will react to and resonate with similar types of energy in the world around them, including the energy running through our body. Crystals can help change or improve that energy. The minerals within each will determine the type and frequency of its vibration, giving it its specific properties. Some crystals are good for conducting electricity and light and are used in manufacturing electronics like cellphones, while others are good at transmitting sound and are used for sonar scans and other tasks.

Quartz has an energy that is great for keeping time, and it's always involved in the creation of watches. Healing crystals react to the different energies inside the body. This is why certain types of crystals will have particular effects on a person, such as blue or green stones that tend to be used for healing. Some crystals radiate strong vibrations that affect the energy in the brain, and having these crystals in a room can influence the mood and state of mind of those near to them. A great benefit is that you don't have to be aware of the crystal for it to work, and even if a visitor in your home thinks it's just a decoration, they can still feel the calming effect of the beautiful blue agate displayed on your mantle.

There are many different ways to use crystals, and some methods are more effective with certain types, but all methods can be effective to some extent. It is, however, very important to have an open mind and positive attitude when using crystals to heal, as a negative mindset will influence the energy in your body and cancel out any positive effects the crystals may have. It's perfectly fine to be a little skeptical and unsure, but with an open mind, you may be pleasantly surprised. If you try crystal healing with the thought "this is stupid and it won't work" strongly in your mind, the crystals won't do you any harm, but they probably won't do you any good either.

Colors in Crystal Healing

As mentioned earlier, the minerals that give crystals their color also often give them their specific powers, and so a crystal's effect can be guessed based upon its color. This isn't an exact science, so the rules aren't set in stone, and there are some crystals that defy them, but this color classification can be a good guideline to work with when buying crystals, especially for beginners. It will take a lot of time and effort to memorize the abilities of each individual crystal, even just the basics.

Below are some basic colors and their healing abilities:

• White and colorless crystals tend to encourage peace and purity, meaning they are useful for cleansing the body and spirit and in creating peaceful vibes in an area or around people wearing these types of crystals. They are usually easy to work and connect with and can sometimes be used to help cleanse other crystals or boost their effects. This color association is quite common and has become a strong symbol in many cultures, such as a white wedding dress or white flag. The most common types of white and colorless crystals are clear quartz, opal, fluorite, moonstone, and white opal.

• Blue crystals tend to have calming effects and can help with communication. These types of crystals can make it easier for people to express themselves and communicate with others. They encourage the ability to speak calmly and express ideas and truths, and they are a good tool to aid you in dealing with other people. Lapis lazuli, amazonite, sapphire, turquoise, and topaz are some of the most commonly known types of blue crystals.

• As with the color in general, green crystals represent growth and life, making them perfect for healing. Green crystals can also be used to help develop and nurture new relationships and can keep you focused on your work. Many green crystals also boost fertility. Good examples of green crystals are emerald, malachite, jade, aquamarine, and peridot.

● Pink crystals help boost romantic emotions and attractions and can help in developing and maintaining romantic relationships. They can also encourage more compassion and kindness in a person. The color pink represents love for a reason, after all. Pink crystals can help you overcome heartache and get rid of emotional baggage. These crystals are also believed to be effective against heart diseases. Your most common pink crystal with these abilities is rose quartz, but rhodonite and pink tourmaline are also good examples.

● Yellow crystals are great for helping you feel good and happy. These crystals encourage positive energy, confidence, optimism, enlightenment, and a better understanding of self. They can also help you perceive things differently. They also bring a sense of warmth and joy into your life. Good examples of yellow crystals are labradorite, citrine, and yellow jasper.

• Orange crystals are ideal for artists, as they boost creativity and confidence and encourage freedom of thought. They can also help support and manage big changes in your life and be useful aids when it comes to making decisions. Many reports and studies have shown them to help in dealing with stomach problems. Carnelian, amber, sunstone, and tourmaline all fit into this category.

• Purple crystals are associated with spirituality and mystic energy. They are best suited to help develop the third eye or to simply help you find new inspiration and purpose by tapping into the divine. Purple crystals are often associated with royalty and strong religious figures and were the most often used in magical rituals throughout many cultures. These crystals are great tools to use for deep relaxation or meditation. The most prominent purple crystals are amethyst, spirit quartz, and lepidolite.

• Red crystals tend to be strong and encouraging. They provide energy and passion, help develop courage, and encourage you to take action. They are great for curing apathy and listlessness and can give you a much-needed boost if you are in a negative emotional state. Many red crystals can also speed up your metabolism and help you burn fat a little more quickly. Ruby, red jasper, and garnet are some of the most popular red crystals.

• Brown crystals help garnish stability and inner energy. They assist in keeping you grounded in a busy, chaotic world and can help you regain and maintain your composure. Brown crystals can also help you feel more at ease and comfortable with your surroundings and help you reconnect with the earth and nature. Brown stones can also help treat ADD. Some of the best examples of brown crystals are tiger's eye, smoky quartz, and bronzite

• Black crystals are the guardians of the crystal world, as they provide a sense of security and protect you from negative energy. They tend to alleviate the fear of physical harm, provide mental fortitude, encourage you to keep negative elements out of your life, and help you connect to the physical world. Many black stones can encourage a sense of well being or make you feel more physically powerful and daring, and they are a great comfort to have with you when you are concerned about your physical safety. They also provide additional healing against immune diseases. Black crystals are also often called barrier crystals because of their protective properties. The best known black crystals are onyx, obsidian, jet, and hematite.

There are many other colors to be found in the crystal world, all with their own traits and abilities, but the majority can be divided into one of the basic color groups mentioned above. In some cases, such as with dalmatian jasper, beryl, and certain types of agate, two or more colors are very prominent, and the crystal will usually have a combination of the abilities associated with those colors. These color groupings are a great factor to think about to help decide where to start with buying healing crystals, but if you have the time for it, it is advised to find out a bit more about the properties and abilities of the specific crystals you are buying.

Shapes in Crystal Healing

Different shapes influence the vibrations of crystals, so crystals are often cut into specific forms that can help boost their potency or alter their abilities. Because of this, shapes have taken on certain meanings within the crystal world.

- Spheres are shapes that radiate the energy of a crystal in all directions. They are good for connecting you with your surroundings, in creating balance, and in boosting abilities that encourage peace and relaxation. This shape is also ideal to use for psychic development and can slow down or prevent harmful or imbalanced energies. This shape is considered to be great for helping develop the third eye. Crystals cut into a spherical shape are often great aids in meditation. The sphere is the most common shape used in crystal scrying.

• Pyramids are considered a sacred shape and have been used to harness power by many civilizations throughout history, with ancient Egyptians being a good example. This type of shape harnesses and amplifies energy tremendously, and crystals cut into this shape have very strong effects. If crystals that encourage energy flow and help channel energy are cut into a pyramid shape, they can be a great tool to boost the abilities of other crystals. Pyramids are a good shape to place around the home and can be a good centerpiece for a crystal grid, as it enhances the entire grid.

• Cube shapes often occur naturally among some crystal types, and this shape tends to have a grounding effect; cubic crystals can help ground and seal natural energy. They also root you to physical plain and are a great shape for crystals with physical type abilities.

• Crystal points and towers are a very common shape for crystals and often occur naturally. These shapes are perfect for manifesting energy and intentions, as well as for directing energy. Many crystals that form natural points are only lightly polished and have the bottom cut off to form a base they can stand on.

• Crystal clusters occur when many crystal points grow together on a single matrix. These clusters direct energy in many different directions and vibrate at a much higher frequency, making their abilities stronger than the same amount of individual crystals. Crystal clusters are absolutely great for displaying around the house as they spread large amounts of energy over a large space, and they are very attractive and fascinating to look at. Admiring a large crystal cluster can sometimes keep you busy for ages.

- Heart-shaped crystals help attract love and affection and connect with our hearts. Small hearts are easy to carry with you, while larger hearts can be strategically placed throughout the house, such as in the bedroom. Almost any type of crystal can be cut into a heart shape, but it is especially effective when combined with crystals that boost feelings of love and attraction.

- Crystals can be cut into faceted or rounded wands which are mainly used in crystal massage. The pointed end of the wand is used to direct the energy through your body and aura, while the wider base can help remove negative energy. These crystals can also be utilized to channel other types of energy.

• Tumbled crystals are best for beginners. They have a smooth, organic shape that radiates energy gently, and the rounded edges make them safe and comfortable to keep directly on the body for a long period of time. They tend to be a bit smaller, which makes it easy to keep them in a bag, in the car, in little bowls all around the house, or tucked under a pillow. Another great benefit of tumbled crystals is that it is the cheapest shape for crystals, making it affordable to obtain a wide variety of crystals to experiment with.

• It often happens that crystals are carved into different sculptures that can have great significance. The specific shape is determined by the purpose and can have corresponding effects. Crystals can be carved into religious symbols to help boost spirituality or into specific animal shapes to connect with spirit animals. Crystals cut into yin and yang shapes can help provide balance in life. Crystal skulls are deeply connected to myth and lore and are believed to encourage healing. Many believe that angel-shaped crystals can help you connect to and channel angelic energies. There are hundreds of shapes that crystals can be cut and carved into, each having their own significance and effects.

Crystal Placement

Although placement doesn't have a direct impact on the effects of a crystal, it is important to carefully consider where to put a crystal in your home. Every room in a house has a specific purpose, and the shapes, effects, and abilities of the crystals within a room should mirror that purpose. Crystals with calming effects should be placed in rooms that need peace and quiet, such as a library or study. Crystals that enhance focus and determination are more suitable for workplaces, and crystals that improve communication and provide relaxed and comfortable energy are a great addition to dining and living rooms, where guests are usually entertained.

Having a crystal in the wrong place can have undesirable effects. A good example is placing a crystal that boosts intense emotion and provides energy in a baby's bedroom, when crystals with soothing, relaxing, and protective effects would be a better choice. Another thing to consider carefully when placing crystals is the different types of crystals that might end up sharing the same space. Combining crystals by putting them together or close to each other can be a great way to manage their abilities and effects in a space with more precision, and wonderful things can happen when you have the right crystal combinations. Unfortunately, bad combinations are also a possibility, and the energies in different crystals can clash with one another and have a negative effect, or they can completely cancel each other out and render each other virtually useless.

Chapter 4: Healing Gemstones & Crystals

Over the years, holistic healers have taken advantage of the mystical and medicinal qualities inherent in gemstones and crystals. Whether it is to achieve balance or well-being for themselves and their customers or to cure their chakras. Healing gemstones are, however, no longer just for natural healers! Most people start to take in their own hands the influence of gemstones. But, how do you select the crystals or gemstones that are perfect for you?

It may be difficult to find gemstones for your needs, but once you know their background and power, it is easy to select the right gemstones. The main use of gemstones and crystals has been for medicinal and religious reasons throughout history. During these days, however, gems are considered rare. It makes them available to a small few. Thankfully, nowadays, everyone who needs them is more readily accessible.

Several people are skeptical about the powers of gemstones. Nevertheless, modern science also acknowledges the powers of gemstones and crystals. You don't learn they're used in watches, lasers, computers and even important applications. Because of this encouragement for medicine, we still have their ability to promote actual treatments in the body to demonstrate and distinguish.

Gems and crystals all have varying degrees of magnetic strength. Many of them are extremely beneficial to the use of human form treatment. We are known to emit small vibrations and frequencies which can influence our life. Jemes are used for healing, shaping, changing and combining mind and soul in many different religions and traditions. It is often used to trigger our abilities in many different respects to sooth, relax, cure and balance.

But many people still have to learn the healing practices of gemstones and crystals given the abilities of gemstones. Some of the first things you need to learn about gems are how to purify them from previous energies.

The gem should be washed by leaving them for six to eight hours under running water. And it can also be buried overnight in the soil (withdrawn afterward, of course!). You can otherwise put them over a candle's flame until it melts. When your gemstone is polished, it should be put in the direct sunlight for purification, as it is a marvelous source of energy.

Note, your stones should be wearing. You don't have much use to lie in a jewelry box. A healing gemstone will help you heal both your mind and spirit at all times with little or no effort. Just being in balance with the stone and letting it function, its power is enough for your body.

Once you are committed to looking for knowledge of healing gemstones, you need an open mind and heart. There are many different theories about why and how gemstones work, but some can be confused or jaded with time. Only trust in the stones and allow the energy to work through the magic of its own.

Whether you are a beginner in the world of healing stones or an old soul only looking for new rocks. You can choose from several different gemstones or crystals. Some of the most common stones and their skills are not so well known.

Rose Quartz is one of the most common healing gemstones. It is renowned for its gentle healing powers, primarily used for his possibilities of healing the soul. It is used to protect the heart from physical pain to psychological heartbreak therapy.

It is also a gift to those who need to understand how to love themselves.

Fluorite: another common gemstone community stone. Though available in many different colors, it is a stone that can help protect someone from negativity. In short, this stone absorbs and helps to keep negative energy nearby. Also, you will need to clean up the stones, which are known to absorb negative energy, at least once a week.

Lapis: a top dog in the gemstone world. It's said to help release mysteries. It is often used to help users with frustration and emotional barriers.

Hematite: a building stone many uses. It is unmistakable in silver-gray metallic coloring for any other gemstone. It is often used as an instrument for people who want to avoid earthly activities or events by quitting their bodies.

Amethyst: this beautiful purple stone is often connected to spiritual cure. It is known to help its clients to become more aware and intelligent.

Jade: Used to teach acceptance through soothing energy. It is used to motivate someone to make himself and others less important.

Turkish: used literally for jewelry elegance. It is a rock that can be used to teach. It is a stone often used for meditation or dream experiences.

Cyanite: is used by skilled gemstone healers. It is best used by wearing this near the chakra of the neck. It is used as a focal point for the canalization and opening of contact centers. A brilliant rock, unlike many other gemstones, can cleanse itself from negative energies.

Citrine: another front runner in the gemstone world. It's a lovely yellow stone that helps manifest your goals. It can help to draw plenty and personal strength.

Obsidian: is used again as a defensive agent or grounding agent. It is known to help to bring about change, serenity, and clarity.

Amazonite: a gemstone used to boost the quality of oneself.

Amber: Used to remove stress heaviness. This helps joy to reach your life again.

Apatite: Another stone often used for contact in your country. It is used when an incomprehension occurs and can help calm any tension that emerges from a war.

Green Aventurine: used for physical treatment. It is worn over the body's distressing portion.

Blue Aventurine: Used to improve blood circulation.

Coral: used as an emotional basis.

Diamond: Not just the best friend of a woman! It is used for social clarification.

Emerald: for physical and emotional care. This is by far one of the best healing elements to date.

Carnelian: A tool used to improve imagination and cognitive process. * Carnelian.

Grey Moonstone: used as a focus for other stones which allow you to use their energies and the energy of the moonstone.

Moss Agate: used as a starting stone in meditation to touch mother nature herself.

Mexican onyx: is used to cure sleep disorders and insomnia.

Black opal: this stone will allow the body and mind to focus.

Ruby: Often love and romance-related times. It is used to open the heart chakra to let love know.

Sapphire: A lovely rock, known for helping to clear the mind.

Easy Crystal Experiments

We have a fall in the air, assume. We'll see a cool and smooth drop of water if we look closely. If the microscope is shot and magnified around 2000 times (it's now 40 meters long and large size of the classroom) and looked closely, we'll still see very smooth water, but wiggly artifacts are moving about (paramecia). We could stop here and look for these important parameters, but then we would turn to biology. Let's focus on wind more than that.

Let's magnify the water 2000 times, so the diameter is roughly 15 miles. When we look carefully, we can see how many movements a crowd of Super Bowl fans are arriving at the next exit but it's still boring and hard to see. We will now magnify the magnification by 250 times, so two groups of hydrogen atoms and oxygen atoms are to be seen in a small group like Mickey Mouse (total magnification of about one billion times). This small atom group is known as a molecule.

The photo on the right is rather optimized; but above all, the real picture dances and wiggles, watching it magnified 1 billion times. The picture on the right is rather perfect. The explanation this picture is not perfectly correct is because the atoms, in the same manner as magnets, are joined together like glue. Yet they repel them, unlike objects if these atoms are squeezed too closely together.

The motion is what we refer to as air. If the temperature rises (say fluid on the hot stove), the jiggles increase and there will be a greater distance between the atoms.

Suppose we lower our waterfall temperature now, we note decreases in jiggling motion and the atoms are fused to a new model known as ice at very low temperatures. Interestingly, the solid form of each atom (crystalline array) is located. Water is one of the only molecules strengthened by expansion. The ice crystal pattern is shown (right)—many pants are included. When atoms jiggle faster than normal, the open structure breaks off (melt) to cover the gaps with rising temperatures (and jig).

What's the size of a nuclear? The size of the atoms in orange is around the size of the original orange if orange is lifted to the size of the Earth.

Crystals are formed either by solidification (think of your freezer's ice crystal) or by "rising" (as we are going to pursue home school science). There is one very unique solution for the manufacture of Kristal. This is known to be a "supersaturated solid solution." What does this mean? What does this mean? An example here: when you continuously add salt to the cup of the water through the containers, the salt does not vanish (dissolve) anymore and produces a lump and a spoonful. You will find out more about crystalline development.

The point in which a lump starts to form is just beyond the point in which a solution is saturated. The lump disappears when the saltwater gets heated. Now you can use more and more salt until it can no more salt (you're going to see another lump rising in the ground). Now it's a super-saturated style. Fill the lump with a little air. Remove. Your crystal-growth solution is packed. But what happens to this?

Now you can grow crystals if you add something to the crystals, such as a rock or a pin. Once you seed the object, they begin to form quicker (coat it with the things you have been forming with, like salt or sugar).

Speedy crystal tips: if you keep the solution cold, crystals will grow faster. Use the highest position of your room, heating pad, or box with a lit lamp.

When you apply too much salt (or some other solids) and you get an enormous rock that you can not extract from the bowl, you will crystalize the solution at the same time. If you have too little salt, you will wait forever for crystals to grow. To find the best way to mix it takes time and patience.

Geodes A geode is a crystallized mineral deposit that, before opening it, is normally very bland and ordinary outdoors! An eggshell is used to mimic a lava gas bubble. You are left with a geode by dissolving the aluminum into the water and putting it on the eggshell (in real life, it's a pocket of the bubble). (Make sure your eggshells are clean. (Note: those crystals don't eat, just look.) Start a small cup of warm water and dissolve the most alum possible in the water to create a saturated solution (i.e., if you add some more alum not dissolve, it will just fall to the ground). Fill the eggshells with the solution and hold. Remember that the solution will evaporate in the next couple of days. You have a DIY geode if the solution is completely evaporated. You have too much water and little aluminum when you have not formed crystals.

Gemstones Complete the above solution in a clean glass jar and leave for 2 days. Squeeze and save later. Save. Keep crystals! Hold crystals! Hold crystals! Keep crystals!

Filler with an additional saturation solution in another glass jar and hang the crystal onto the jar lid by a string (the experiment above). Raise it for a few days and wait. The crystallization process needs to be used to produce candy. You should make a supersaturated sugar solution and use this solution to create your home-made candy crystals. (Seed the string for fast growth.) The largest amount of sugar dissolved in the liquid is a supersaturated solution. Boil the rock candy in a large pot on the stove three cups of water. Mix eight cups of sugar and mix one cup at a time (if we didn't heat the water, we'd just wind it in a soaking solution. Yellowish and thick should be the liquid. Turn off the heat and let it stay 4 hours (or less than 120 degrees F). Add a few drops of food color (for decorative crystals) in the clean glass containers of sugar water solution. Hold a string on a skewer and place the skewer horizontally across the bowl's mouth.

A water jelly crystal can grow more than 300 times its size when hydrated (added liquid) (through a part of the hardware store's garden usually "Soil Moist"). Together with each cup half a cup of water. Add a few drops of food colored and blend. Remove a few crystals and you have to stand for 20 minutes. With your hand, squish them! Squish your hands at them! In an empty water bottle combine a variety of different colors (within layers) and show the colors blend. Make a big rainbow wall of fluorescent plastic pipe housing. (Test layers of black, white, red and orange and green from nowhere!). Place them on a towel and allow to dry for a few days to reuse crystals (they can stain under the towel, so you can add a layer of paper).

Salt Stalactite Take a mixed solution from the warm water and the Epsom salts. (Fill in two empty glass jars with a salt solution to prevent a further breakdown when you add more). On a foil layer or cookie sheet, put the bottles. Move from a jar to a jar the thread or rope. Wait with impatience for three days. A stalactite must develop from the middle of the string!

Crystal Orgone and Generator How to Use Together with Quantum Physics Laws

The mixture of quantum physics and orgone technology improves health/richness and happiness.

Quantum Physics tells us that we construct our truth through what we think. Our thoughts are building our future. If we want health/wealth and happiness, then we must feel that way. The problem is that such feelings can't be kept alive for a long time.

We can use the science of orgone generators to keep our feelings alive in the Quantum Ocean until they manifest themselves in our lives.

The Ond Orgone Generator is a device like this. This solid orgone generator is based on five DT crystals.

Open all the noises in your room. It enables you to earn money. Clear your mind about the noisy and vibrating telephones, ELF poles, TV and computer noise. It helps you find peace of mind and adapt the psychological patterns of your body to nature.

When Orgone generates life force, it is a simple radionic unit.

A radionic device activates the direct transfer of energy from the everlasting limitless store, now called the Quantum Ocean (God's mind). This force of life is moduled to a destination—YOU through therapy (symbol, radionics, photo, etc.).

Life forces have many names such as Prana, Chi, Mana, Ond, Odic and Animal Magnetism, etc. The movements of two areas of the body produce LifeFORCE equally. It is very much like moving two cups through a magnetic field — electricity is produced. It is very similar to the passage of two copper wire parts through a magnetic field. The process and orgone use equivalent amounts of COPPER BB 'S and NON-METALIC RESIN. The other one repels it.

The PUSH–PULL of life force fields creates extra life force. The CRYSTAL in the COPPER COIL produces an Earth-resonant harmonic frequency pulse generator.

A sacred geometrical shape, the CONIC PYRAMID creates space for the interaction of life force fields. The output waves are modulated as well. A person close to the Ond Orgone Device draws the energy of this life into his aura. This strength of existence is also derived from an individual's STRUCTURE relation (hair, blood, or picture). Any dangerous EMF motion past the Ond Orgone Generator is positive strength in life.

On the physical plane of existence, energy, magnetism, gravity, elven waves, mobile telephones, radioactivity, etc. are all abstract forces. We all send vibrations. Some of these people's sounds are harmful to people. Wilhelm Reich called DOR (Deadly Orgone). As the array is square, the amplitude of these EMF forces decreases. The power of life is subjective, but also stronger. It is not made by people and can even be directed mentally. The major shamans, medicine men, and curators used their minds to heal and mutilate. Some sensitive people can feel this energy.

This life force does not move like EMF waves across 3D space. It moves through STRUCTURAL LINKs through hyperspace. The stronger the link, the the the flow of life force.

EXAMPLE: If energy is transferred to a strand of your body via a radionic device, life force is applied to you regardless of length. It is the similarity of objects that defines life force movement instead of physical distance. Because your hair (DNA) is the same structure because your body (DNA), your life force travels quickly. HEALING begins, WEALTH starts moving towards you, HAPPINESS starts inside.

MENTAL RADIONICS MAGIC is a representation of a human-minded life force throughout the ages. Wizards, shamans, and healers have all the force of will in integrating mental forces to maintain these spiritual processes. Today, we don't have this discipline, we need assistance.

The Ond Orgone machine is a simple tool for radionics, which enables all of us to be modern magicians. It provides an intense quality of life. We only have to offer the signs of healing and the target.

HARMFUL EMF WAVES HARMFUL Life strength comes from the interaction of two Life Force forces. The ond orgone system provides power lines, cell phones, computers, TVs with DOR or EMF waves. Once you reach your home, ELF towers will serve as the second field. The relationship between these two fields will create another good strength of life.

The DOR field is therefore absorbed through the Orgone process. The system will be very close to how air cleaner functions at home. It's also like a tree's bad air and good wind.

The Orgone Generator acts as a basic radionic tool, where you can attract safety, prosperity, and happiness with the right symbols. I like the runes. I like the runes. I like the runes. I like the runes. It also helps clear your home from dangerous DOR waves.

Wilhelm Reich has shown the energy matrix that absorbs and captured Orgone energy, mixing organic materials (plastic resin, soil, wool, cotton, etc) with a metal component. Organic compound (plastic, water, wood, wool, etc.). (LIFE-FORCE) By adding a' Crystal' to the combination due to its intrinsic character, you can now customize your and orgone device. You may mentally program the crystal to channel the orgone energy to a certain mission, purpose or desire. The Ond Orgone Machine is a simple radionics machine. Radio equipment generates and transmits orgone energy for one reason. The conical pyramid (Sacred Geometrical Solid) provides a working matrix in the "DOR" (deadly orgone energy) into constructing orgone energy for the Ond Orgone Generator.

As everything that we see was first created in Quantum Ocean or Mind Of God, we can use your mental and cognitive energy power to enhance the work of our Ond Orgone Generator. Loading or coding your Orgone Generator with your mental power for one particular purpose: maintain the Orgon Machine before your Solar Plexus in both hands. You can either sit down or stand. Take a deep breath and inhale your head into this creative universal healing power (hyperphysical gland).

Attempt this: breathe the spirals of pure, sparkling, fantastic Sunlight into your pocket with your Orgone Generator. Remember that the Sun shines everywhere, even at night. The sun is the highest source of artistic and healing power for our lives to co-create our visions and shape our lives. Breathe in this exquisite spiraling energy and ask yourself mentally, "In every cell of my physical, mental and spiritual life I now live in the mystical, creative and healing forces. Hold this incredible energy inside yourself with your eyes shut down. Then, as you exhale very slowly, pour out this force from your Third eye (the pineal gland in your forefront)."How long do you need to use the Orgone method and your pineal hypophysis to tell your life what you want, how broad is the curtain of negative programming? What programming have you accepted in your midst? Programming ends the pace of your life of wealth, stability, health, and happiness?

Light Crystal Display

The use of liquid crystals has been a breakthrough in screen design and numerous display applications including watches, television and cell phones. The old CRT monitor was big and bulky while the use of liquid crystals in every pixel made it possible to look at displays and display systems slimmer and smarter. LCD monitors are also electrical efficient, as LCD monitors require minimal energy consumption, and can also be operated using batteries instead of having monitors that use a large amount of energy. This is why it is very flexible and can be used on various mobile phones.

There are distinctive numbers of pixels and fixed-pixel images in LCD screens. More easily, LCD monitors have a native resolution or a certain pixel density that shows a certain resolution. The screen resolution or pixel size informs consumers of the ability of the computer to show an image clearly. All LCD screens of the same size display the same resolution as all LCD monitors, regardless of the brand they are. If a different resolution is put outside of the native resolution, extrapolation may occur, allowing multiple pixels to produce the same image causing a dull screen. Buyers must be told that buying large LCD monitors leads to smaller image displays in practice, which is one of those cases in which larger monitors are smaller.

The purchasing of an LCD screen is a cost-effective decision on the part of the consumer. The benefits of LCD control are far superior to the very low specific considerations. LCD monitors produce less radiation than cathode-ray tube monitors or CRT monitors because there is no build-up of energy on its back. It is very easy on the eyes and it is much less painful and frustrating to deal with. This contains no phosphorus and will not cause photo burns during long breaks. Apart from its sleek and elegant appearance, LCDs are very cheap and budget-friendly, they can also minimize monthly electricity consumption as they use less power when they are used or stand-by. When buying LCDs, pick the ones that are suitable for your screen resolution requirements. Although it is tempting to have massive widescreen monitors, check to see how they look when you open websites and documents to see if they are appropriate for your requirements. Please ask for energy-saving tools to save more on your bills.

What to think when buying an LCD screen Most consumers go through Liquid Crystal Display Monitors and have a set of questions. Most consumers want to upgrade their computer monitors, but most still hesitate to buy them. This is mainly due to the many things you need to remember when buying an LCD screen. Despite popular belief, LCD screens are not costly, in reality, they could even cost as much as if you purchased your old CRT monitor first. It's also pretty much a money saver, so you get real value for your money. To explain the impressive capabilities of LCD screens, a list of the most frequently asked questions about them and their responses is available.

What is the aboriginal resolution?

The display screen dimensions are shown in pixels (e.g. 1024x768). CRT displays have different pixel counts, but LCDs only have one value or number of pixels, regardless of what product they are, if they are in equal sizes. This ensures that every LCD screen has a defined resolution that customers must consider because they must comply if they want the best results. Bigger LCDs would mean that the images shown are much smaller while smaller screens display larger images.

What does the aspect ratio mean?

The aspect ratio is the ratio between the number of horizontal and vertical pixels. Some screens have 4:3 aspect ratios. Nevertheless, modern LCD screens have aspect ratios of up to 16:10, and LCD screens can even have high-definition features of up to 16:9 while ultra-wide displays have an impressive aspect ratio of 2:1. It displays the far more detailed image quality and contrast capabilities of an LCD screen.

What is the time for a response?

To display color or an object in a specific area of the screen, the liquid crystals need to transfer the electric current through the LCD panels. The time it takes for the current to pass through the panels and the time required to change it, turn on or off by liquid crystals is referred to as the response time. Response time not only applies to on or off the screen, but also to light objects and gray and black backgrounds displayed. In general, the response time of LCD monitors is quite slow. The rising time or the time it takes to turn on is very fast but the falling time or the time it takes to turn off is a little bit slower that is why you will notice a short blur when images suddenly shift to bright streaks on the monitor with a dark background. This is especially important when you buy an LCD screen for gaming.

What is the point of view?

The pixel shows the corresponding color, as the electric current passes through the LCD panel. But the image displays the shadow immediately in front of the audience right before the screen. This LCD screen feature does not permit clear images when viewing the display at the side or any angle other than directly in front of the monitor. Although it requires a simple view, this feature is popular, particularly if customers would like more privacy with their display. This is also a good reason why consumers often choose dual widescreen displays.

What is luminosity?

Brightness is the monitor's ability to radiate light and color screen. Most of the new screens are very white. It helps the eyes of the consumers to be relaxed with longer use. New LCDs have sophisticated brightness control functionality. The change of creativity depends on the personal choice of the consumer. With an extremely luminous screen, it can be good at times, but it can be bad especially when the ambient light is weak. New LCDs can change the brightness of the screens automatically through sensors and can, therefore, be very useful to use them.

Is the quality of the picture important?

Sure, purchasing LCD screens means getting the best images and videos. The best images on your screen and the ease with which LCD screens have on your eyes is, by far, one of the most appealing things to purchase. Since the CRT monitor size of your image displays is quite small, LCD screens offer customers accurate, crisp and transparent images due to their very large range of looks and resolutions, from widescreen to high-definition features that show life-like images. LCD monitors ' image quality is undoubtedly one of the main reasons why customers love them at first sight.

The future of computer monitors, and other display systems is buying advice on LCD screens. The advantages and features of the latest generation of monitors are obvious. Try before you buy while shopping for screens. Tell the technician to disable it before you purchase it. View pictures on your computer or try to open the web pages and documents you frequently imagine or open at home and see if the photo view is right for your eyes. Test the screen's luminosity and try different sizes. Every size has a different resolution so make sure you find one that best suits you. If you need to replace the old CRT then why not go out and buy the best, try HD monitors and I'm sure you'll be delighted by the results. You must also find an immobilizing screen. The amount of space you can work with on your computer is to monitor real estate. Many desktops display larger images but show less real-estate screen. Wouldn't you like to see apps and sites overpopulating your screen, right? Check the immobilization display and see whether you have enough space to view pages and applications without having to scroll through papers like a mile long. I suggest you go for dual screens if you certainly need a lot of space. Dual screens make your desk look cool and create more screen space to work comfortably. Dual LCD screens are the way to fulfill all your needs for multiple tasks. Check for screens with USB ports on the arm. For USB ports, performance and availability can be improved. This is particularly helpful when most ports are in the CPU below your chair. You can also use built-in speakers to check displays. The speakers will accentuate your existing audio equipment and create a round sound sensor environment. Check the newest models with most accessories and features when shopping for screens.

Chapter 5: Color Power

Crystals are not only grouped according to the months that they represent. They are also grouped according to the color that they have and each color has a specific meaning as well as a specific chakra point that they work best with. This is done in order to help a crystal healer discern what kinds of crystals to use for a specific ailment and sickness. With no further ado, let us look into the different color groups of crystals and these groups mean.

The crystals in the red group are crystals that help in energizing, activating and stimulating the body's systems because the color red is associated with the terms such as sparkle and ignition and life. They are linked with the first chakra, which involves the spinal cord that is mainly responsible for mobility and action. Because of the rejuvenating color of the red crystals, their main purpose is to give energy. Examples of the crystals in the red group include amethyst and ruby.

When you mix the colors red and white together, you will get the end result of pink which is a color the gives off a subtle and gentle effect to the body. The crystals in the pink group are the crystals that are associated with the heart chakra and these crystals help bring in an emotional side to our actions and decisions. They also help a person feel calm and composed during difficult times. They are the perfect mix of white light and energy.

Red and yellow, if equally mixed, results to the color of orange. The crystals in the orange group are the best crystals that have both the properties of focus and energy. These crystals are affiliated with the second chakra or the chakra that dictates if there is a flow of energy or lack thereof in the body.

The solar plexus chakra which is responsible for the regulation of the nervous system's functions, the localization and identification of the things around us and the functioning of the body's immune and digestive system is associated with the crystals in the yellow group.

The crystals in the green group are linked to the heart chakra. These crystals help in balancing emotions and encouraging feelings and relationships that are beneficial to one's personal growth.

When it comes to communication, the crystals belonging to the light blue group will be of much help to you because they are associated with the throat chakra. The vibrations of the light blue crystal help in making your communication skills, both inter and external, more articulate and refined.

The color of the indigo is associated with the brow chakra or the "third eye" chakra. The crystals under the indigo group can help in sharpening one's intuition, perception and comprehension.

The crown chakra, which is situated at the topmost of the head, is affiliated with the colors of the violet group. The crystals from this group can maintain the homeostasis between extremes. They can also help in improving imagination, inspiration and empathy.

Another group of crystals that are associated with the crown chakra is the white group of crystals. Crystals bearing the color of white reflects the feeling of clarity, universality cleanse and purification.

If white stones reflect light, the crystals in the black group absorb the light that is why they have the blackish color. The crystals belonging to this group are used in purification and making potentials visible.

The crystals belonging to the multicolored group are the ones that are used for multi purposes and have rainbow fractures.

Since they reflect a wide variety of colors, they are able to reflect a wide variety of effects and qualities too, making them versatile to fit into any purpose.

These are the different kinds and different groups of crystals according to color. Knowing them and mastering them will be very beneficial in choosing the right and relevant crystal that you will use in order to heal.

Chapter 6: The Healing Power Of Crystals Do They Work?

Created over millennia, healing crystals bring life to the components of the Earth and the universe. Harnessing the energy of the Sun, Moon and oceans, the gemstones unite us with the Universe once we interact with them. Many individuals ask if the crystals have spiritual capabilities and while many tales depict the healing stones' impacts, it depends on your knowledge. Not every individual is capable of understanding crystal mending and it takes a deep level of consciousness to open your mind and soul to the practice, but once you start, the journey sprinkled with alluring, mysterious and particular crystals will thrill you.

People either believe in the healing characteristics of crystals, or they think it's as probable to operate as collecting rock from the floor and attempting to do magic.

The healing forces and methods to use them may seem like magic, but crystals have a scientifically sound history. While crystals are still seen as an option in healing, the explanation of why crystals do what they do truly sounds very logical. Undoubtedly, crystals oscillate at their frequency, just as body cells and your Chakras resonate with them. This implies that when we come into touch with crystals, these distinct frequencies fulfill and improve your physical, spiritual and mental equilibrium.

Crystals enclose the impressive ability to convert, absorb, augment and conduct energy.

We are energy. We are surrounded by energy in every form and crystals are the perfect conductors. The vibrations of the gemstones change based on the energy type that surrounds them, therefore every rock has a particular and distinct aftermath on each person. Originally, crystal therapy was used to readjust the energy centers known as Chakras and convert the features of the body, developing in this way a pure power range. It is also believed that the ability of crystals does not stop at the spiritual level, but the changes in the energy field also influence and heal the physical body.

What can crystals do for me?

Once you've started using crystals, an excellent method to harness their mending energy is to use healing stones to manifest your plans and what you dream of achieving in life. Regarding crystals, these otherworldly stones link us to the Earth since they are concrete, physical shapes with strong vibrations. This energy remains to link with you when you carry these intentional crystals near to your skin, or when you put them in your setting. With every idea and purpose, these crystals take up your distinctive vibrational energy and amplify the positive vibrations that you cultivate.

In this eerie world of energies, crystal frequency guides you on your trip because it enables you to find your purpose and reminds you of your attachment to Earth. The well believed out purpose is the starting point for healing crystals because the particular motives instilled in your regular habits of thought are also component of their energy.

Why do crystals work?

Clear Quartz existed since the beginning of time and ancient populations have used crystals as protective talismans, peace gifts and jewels. Today, glass represents 12% of the Earth surface and is used in almost every kind of industry, including timekeeping, electronics, data storage and more. If crystals interact through computer chips, then isn't it feasible that this vibrational energy could be converted in other forms? Furthermore, with their bond to the planet and their life-giving components, it is reasonable that crystals are widely healing, particularly since they left their mark in almost every precedent civilization.

Among the first bits of scientific proof concerning the strength of crystals is the research performed by IBM scientist Marcel Vogel. While observing crystals develop under a microscope, he realized that their shape had taken the form of anything he was talking about. He assumed that these shocks are the consequence of the continuous assembling and disassembling of bonds between molecules. He also evaluated the metaphysical strength of quartz crystal and demonstrated that stones could store ideas comparable to how recordings use magnetic energy to record noise.

Albert Einstein said that everything around us is energy and just like sound waves, your ideas match the sensations of everything that is manifested in your lives.

Therefore, if you confide in the healing capacity of crystals, the positive energy of these rocks will deepen your faith.

Anytime, we can choose our ideas and, as we proceed on our trip, each day provides us with fresh difficulties and beautiful experiences. Healing crystals remind us to silence our thoughts while reconnecting to the mending energy of the Earth. Patience is a valuable experience to gather from crystals because just like the years it took for these gemstones to emerge and mold, learning to work with the power of crystals is also a long process. As you study, develop and grow, use them as a reminder to be thankful for the prosperity offered to you by Mother Nature and the enigmas of the Cosmos.

How do I choose a crystal?

Mending stones have been used since primordial times, so there is an abundance of information and experience passed down from generation to generation.

Once you understand the principles of crystals, the best way of choosing the correct healing stones for your trip is by using your intuition. Specialists claim that the crystal is the one choosing you and not vice versa. Walk around the space and see the crystals that stand out from you. Whether it's the dazzling colors or the otherworldly shapes and patterns that draw you in, every crystal has a unique vibrational energy that works to clear blockages and ward off negative energy.

Finding the correct rock is like any wellness exercise. It needs patience while you're stilling your mind and realigning your mind/body equilibrium. Hold the rock in your palm and think softly about your aim. Notice if you feel emotions such as hot or cold, pulsation, or stillness and quietness. These are all indications that this specific gem is the perfect fit for your spirit.

It also helps to define a specific issue or challenge that you are presently experiencing. If you have difficulty focusing, Fluorite helps to clear up mental and emotional distress that can discourage concentration. To attract abundance, citrine enables you to express your thoughts by conducting the positive energy of the Sun. Carnelian is a strong crystal that allows creative juices to flow.

If you have trouble letting go of old ideas that no longer serve you, Black Turmaline is a strong gemstone for releasing unwanted models that may have transformed into poor practices. It might help you release all the bad vibes from your body and your environment. This stone also acts as a security talisman, which is crucial if you are an individual who can quickly pick up on other people's energy. Hematite is good for deflecting the harmful energies of others by helping you settle and resuscitating your essence using Earth's energy.

If you're looking for a more peaceful life, amethyst is one of the finest motivation crystals to comfort you and restore your equilibrium. Another gemstone that facilitates balancing your emotions is the moonstone, which provides you with assistance when you feel overly emotional or disconnected from your feelings. Rose quartz is also valuable for spiritual well-being because it closes and readjusts the heart Chakra, which amplifies self-esteem and the unreserved love of others.

Whether you're looking for crystals for aesthetic purposes or for attracting peace and tranquility to your lives, they're all working to raise your energy. If you feel comfortable holding the crystal in your palm or touching your skin, get prepared for the chance to rock with this old healing art.

What is an intention?

Reflections generate fluctuations throughout the universe, making setting intentions a strong instrument for attaining happiness and well-being. Having a definite objective gives us understanding into our ambitions, aspirations and principles. Besides, it empowers us to live in the present moment instead of being caught up in negative thinking habits. Intents are like magnets. They're attracting what makes them come true. Setting an intention is a strong instrument to achieve happiness. Creating an objective starts by setting goals that are aligned with your beliefs, ambitions and objectives.

☐Decide what's important to you. Your principles are driving activities in your lives and you will need to acknowledge what counts to you if you wish to be fulfilled.

☐Explore regions of your lives that need to be upgraded. Consider how you can enhance your relationship, career, personal lives, spirituality, wellness and society.

☐ Be specific about what you plan on doing, when you want to do it and why.

☐Bring your intentions back to life. Some of the procedures explained in the next sections will invite you to write them down. Be sure to write them in the present tense as if they're going to happen now and only confirm what you want. It is important to write down your objective too, the aftermath of what you want to depict. Put the sensation in it!

I have my crystal. Now how do I behave?

One of the essential (and often ignored) elements to work with healing crystals is defining your intent or priority. Otherwise stated, you must assign a target to your crystal! Stones try to work for you, but you must guide them. During hard times, when you vibrate at low frequency, your thoughts can float out of the window. When you reconnect with your scheduled crystal, it will assist you in remembering your objectives and limitless possibilities.

The programming of your crystal is easy. Begin by cleaning up your crystal. You can choose your chosen wiping technique and what the most resonates with you. Immerse your crystal in the smoke of a burnt sage stick, Frankincense resin or Copal incense. Place your crystal under the sunlight or the full moon light for a couple of hours (I would suggest at least four). Bury it and let it recharge with Earth's energy. If it's a tiny crystal, you can position it on top of a translucent quartz crystal or a selenite one to purify it and clean up any stuck energy.

Next, keep your crystal in your fingers, near your eyes, take three profound breaths. Think about your faith, the earth and something that brings you happiness. This is going to bond you with your greatest vibration. Your highest vibration may be identified with a religious or sacred belief, a divine figure, or simply a power greater than you. Or it may be linked to a science connection— zero-point power. You're deciding what to call it. Then, while in this mindset of peace and light, pray for your crystal to be freed of any unwanted energy or prior programming.

5 simple ways to use crystals

If you're starting to use crystals, begin with these five strong and vital crystals of intent to foster equilibrium, harmony and peace of mind.

Clear Quartz and How to Use it

One of the most common crystals among beginners, transparent quartz additionally deepens your desire, making it the main element of a crystal collection. It's also the most flexible rock because it amplifies the motions of the rocks around it. Transparent quartz rods are usually used to clean and re-energize crystals. This is due to its strong purification impacts and the capacity to counteract adverse energy blockages.

Sit silently with a rock and think that its white light fills your flesh with beneficial energy. Contemplate your desire for the healing crystal and believe in the strength of its vibrations over the millennia harnessed from Earth.

Selenite and How to Use it

Selenite is another strong cleaning stone because it guarantees a favorable stream of vibrations between your body and other crystals in your collection, making it a perfect crystal for beginners.

Quickly extract adverse energy from your body and clear the aura around you by shifting selenite from your head to your toes. Repeat this purification routine for as long as you need to feel rejuvenated by positive vibrations. After that, you will enjoy a renewed feeling of equilibrium and the security of the white light that links you to the universe.

Shungite and How to Use it

One of the rarest rocks on Earth, Shungite includes antioxidants that give it powerful healing characteristics, including safety from dangerous substances that are detrimental to the body. Shungite is generally utilized to soothe anxiety and accelerate the detoxification process. This healing stone has strong physical impacts, so it's best to bring it gently.

Position a fragment of Shungite right next to your laptop, wi-fi hub, or other electronic devices in your house. We also suggest that you place a bit of Shungite on your cell phone to reduce the impacts of EMFs.

Amethyst and How to Use it

Known for its strong spiritual characteristics, the lovely amethyst is the perfect stone to decorate your house. This visually striking rock is also a great meditation tool because it enhances internal power and offers spiritual security.

As you focus on your purpose, position amethyst in your cabinet or dormitory to exhale calming energies and invitation in abundance. This stone also operates as a supplementary therapeutic instrument for yoga and meditation.

Citrine and How to Use it

Citrine harnesses the energy originated from the Sun. This rock is covered with light, making it ideal for placing it in the windowsill. Its regular infusions of natural light restore and regenerate its strong vibrations. Considered to be one of the strongest rocks for expression, citrine is essential for beginners, since it helps to transform your goal into reality. It also infuses a favorable perspective and stimulates the mind in such a way that you are encouraged to develop healthy practices and be always packed with optimism.

Position a fragment of citrine (we recommend a citrine point) close to your list of dream manifestations to make them come true much faster.

Not only are they brilliant eye candy, but these rocks also bring us back to Mother Earth and her incredible wealth. In the old art of crystal healing, gemstones rock when it gets to good vibrations!

Chapter 7: 50 Crystals To Know (From A To Z)

Aegirine

This stunningly elegant gemstone is black to dark green in colour and is known to possess extremely strong protective energies. By guarding the wearer's chakra network, aura, and physical body in times of danger and difficulty Aegirine has earnt its reputation of instilling confidence, conviction and courage in those affected by its cool, light-hearted energy. Usually found in Canada, Greenland, Russia, Scotland, and Nigeria, Aegirine as a name is derived from the Norse sea god Aegir and has also been called Acmite after the Greek word meaning 'point' which is an apt description as Aegirine is commonly found sticking out of rock, looking not unlike blades protruding from the earth itself. Aegirine is a great crystal for overcoming self-consciousness and the unnecessary shame that comes from facing the overzealous judgements of others of our appearance and/or lifestyle choices.

Agate

Agate is a name commonly used to cover many different varieties of Chalcedony which display an almost endless array of colours, pure, banded, mixed or colourless. Sometimes called the 'earth rainbow' it is said that Agate and its vast colour spectrum is the gemstone embodiment of the varying states of our innermost world. Agate possesses a lower vibrational frequency than most gemstones, however, its energy is extremely influential in balancing the aura, has a stabilising effect which promotes responsibility, reliability, maturity, and also acts as an amazing conduit for spiritual energies which leads to thoughts of self-encouragement and feelings of self-confidence.

Amazonite

Amazonite is a much-loved stone which displays deep shades of turquoise and green and upon first contact is believed to calm the spirit and replenish the soul. Sometimes known as 'The Stone of Truth and Courage' Amazonite empowers the individual along a journey of self-discovery leading to the discovery of one's personal truths. Its calming energy tempers wayward emotions promotes self-control and acts to release any emotional blockages or past traumas that have accumulated within the body's energetic network. Amazonite is great for cleansing and normalising the chakras; it bridges the gap between the physical body and its ethereal counterpart which dissolves inner conflict, focusses efforts and acts amplify results. Amazonite also reinforces and balances the connection between intellect (mind) and intuition (heart) creating a balanced resonance that leads to enhanced abilities and enlightenment.

Amber

Amber has, since Neolithic times been one of the worlds most coveted treasures and not only because for its beautiful warmth of colour which is like golden honey but also because it was looked upon as a gift from the sea. The Greek word Anbar was adopted in the 14th century as the description of what we now call Ambergris (ambergris or grey amber) which is a solid waxy resin-like residue produced by sperm whales and is used in many of the world's most expensive perfumes and fragrances. Somewhere around the 15th century the word amber was extended to include Baltic amber (yellow amber) which is fossilised (usually tree) sap/resin and can take millions of years to form.

Amethyst

Amethyst is a semi-precious type of Quartz crystal found in a number of places around the world and primarily occurs in hues from a light pink/violet to deep purple and blue, sometimes even appearing to have secondary red hues. The name Amethyst comes from the geek word ametusthos which means 'not intoxicated' and throughout history, it has enjoyed the special virtue of preventing drunkenness and overindulgence. It has been said that an Amethyst worn at navel level will bring about soberness and control over indulgent thoughts, whilst keeping Amethyst anywhere on your person could increase intelligence and even inspire shrewd business decisions.

Apatite

Apatite received its name as a derivative of the Greek word meaning 'to deceive', mainly due to the array of different colours in which Apatite chooses to manifest. It is a multi-faceted gemstone that is usually blue but also brown, yellow, and green. Apatite holds several favourable properties such as aiding the body in absorbing calcium which in turn strengthens bones, cartilage, teeth, soothes joints and helps with issues connected to hypertension.

Aquamarine

Getting its name from the Latin aqua Marinus meaning 'water of the sea' Aquamarine has long been worn by sailors for protection while on the water. This calming stone in its hues of blue and green invokes the purity and clarity of crystalline waters with deep connections to trust, truth, and revelation, which when used as a meditation aid can act as a mirror revealing the hidden meanings of reality and even our owns inner depths.

Aventurine

Aventurine crystals are gemstones that contain a healthy amount of Quartz along with other mineral inclusion that acts together to give Aventurine its varying colours. These differing mineral inclusions influence not only the stone's colour but also its inherent energetic attributes, meaningful associations and healing abilities. Its name is derived from the Italian a Ventura meaning 'by chance' and is most commonly associated with luck, regularly known as the 'Stone of Opportunity'.

Bloodstone

The Ancients knew Bloodstone as Heliotrope, a name derived from the two Greek words meaning 'sun-turning' and is said to preserve the mind and body of the wearer and therefore has long been used as a talisman of vibrant health and lasting life. It is a stone known to boost intuition as well as warding off illnesses like colds and flu by invigorating the entire bodily system and may increase overall physical endurance.

Carnelian

Carnelian is a stone found in India as well as South America and exists in red/orange hues with deep red being the most desirable. This stone is a known as one of the stones of motivation and for having strong connections to courage and physical power which can help the shy and introverted in taking on leadership roles and in becoming engaging and eloquent public speakers. The name carnelian comes from the Latin word for 'flesh. In Ancient Egypt, Carnelian was known as 'the setting sun', with its orange form holding female energetic frequencies with the red gemstones being associated with male energies.

Citrine

Citrine's name is derived from the French word citron meaning 'lemon' but is also regularly known as both the Merchant's Stone due to its uncanny ability to increase bank balances, and the Stone of the Mind due to the ancient belief that placing a Citrine stone on the forehead can activate the users latent psychic abilities. Natural Citrine is a pure and radiant yellow, sometimes containing translucent golden hues which emanate energetic frequencies that ground negative energy and create an environment which attracts only the best and most jovial of moods.

Diamond

Otherwise known as the Crystal of Light or the King of Stones, Diamonds are without a doubt the world's best known and most popular gemstone. Diamond has strong connections to winter and as a winter stone with its ice-like colour and clarity, it has a higher energetic frequency than usual, which may explain why it is the hardest mineral on Earth.

Fluorite

Fluorite or the 'Stone of Positivity' for reasons unknown doesn't receive the attention of many of the more popular stones, however, this doesn't make it any the less beautiful or powerful. Fluorite forms in an array of colours and is known as the world's most colourful stone, the most common colour hues include shades of blue and purple, reds, oranges, browns, black, yellows and greens, and clear, and any combination of the above. abilities related to manifestation, creativity, and magic.

Garnet

Garnet is a balancer stone usually found in Africa but also in the United States and Russia, this deep red gemstone has long been a symbol of compassion, love, purity, and truth-giving way to greater levels of spiritual awareness. Garnet exists in a number of forms including the brown/red Almandine (a Stone of Tangible of Truth), Merelini Mint Garnet, and Carbuncle, with the most prized being Noble or Precious Garnet. This highly revered gemstone is known to strengthen the wearer's ability to manifest into being realistic and positive realities within the psychical world around us.

Hematite

Hematite has been in use since at least the time of the ancient Greeks, who used it in the production of rich blood red dyes. The natural Hematite (when polished) displays an iridescent, silvery sheen that is thought to mesmerise the beholder in the same way as moonlight on a clear night. Hematite is an essential addition to any healer's collection. It carries a high iron content thought to improve blood pressure, circulation, promote a healthy heart, and ease menstrual cramps.

Jade

Jade, otherwise known as the 'Dream stone' and holds deep connections to the spiritual world allowing a skilled gemstone user to acquire insights into ancient knowledge both occult and ritualistic (beware-this is not always a good thing). It is another stone that appears to us in a variety of colourful hues with many of them carrying their own individual associations, energies, healing properties and protective qualities but is traditionally assumed to be a green gemstone. Since ancient times it has been said that Jade blesses all that it touches with its energies of purity and serenity.

Kyanite

Kyanite is a blue, green, or black crystal famous for its abilities surrounding high-speed energy transfer, communication, connection, and is perhaps best known for its capacity to enhance psychic abilities like telepathy and divination. This is an essential crystal for healers. The high-frequency energy of Kyanite immediately creates bonds between healer and patient, amplifying the healing effect and speeding up the healing process. It is one of only two crystals that cannot become charged with negative energy by dispelling unwanted adverse energy before any accumulation can take place. This makes it the perfect stone for cleansing other crystals (and rooms) of their unwanted negative energies.

Lapis Lazuli

Lapis Lazuli or 'The stone of Truth' has been in use since at least 4000bc and was in fact used lavishly to adorn King Tutankhamun's sarcophagus. Valued not only for its beauty, Lapis Lazuli was used in the manufacture of the extremely precious and expensive ultramarine dye, medicines and elixirs, and makeup.

Moonstone

Moonstone or 'The Traveller's Stone' has strong associations with and the moon and the feminine energy it represents. Usually, an opaque white at times with a silvery sheen Moonstone can also display beautifully subtle and exquisite hues of pale blue, peach, and grey. Moonstone has been used in jewellery for thousands of years and all over the world and has for the longest time been associated with hope, love, and reconciliation. Emotionally and spiritually Moonstones helps one in overcoming matters of the ego and reduces reliance on, and attachment to unnecessary materialism. It is said that

Moonstone cure insomnia, sleepwalking, sleep paralysis and other conditions concerned with sleep.

Obsidian

Traditionally an opaque black gemstone Obsidian's colour can range from darkest black, brown and can carry a number of different mineral inclusions that can appear as white flecks, not unlike snow to incandescent strips of vibrant blue, violet, red, green, and gold. Obsidian has been considered a 'divine stone' for thousands of years and ancient relics, statues, amulets, jewellery and even weapons with razor-sharp Obsidian blades and tools have been found dating back to the Stone-age. Black Obsidian is believed to aid the body in digestion and the purging of toxins, soothe inflammatory conditions, minimise joint pain and arthritis and speeds up the healing process of cuts and bruises. Obsidian also has the ability to absorb airborne pollution and negative energy, however, due to this uncanny ability Obsidian needs to be regularly cleansed by running it under cold water.

Onyx

Traditionally Onyx form in thick black strips followed by thin white stripes but can display hues of red, brown and honey. Onyx is one of the few stones known for being a 'stone of bad luck' however this has not caused it to fall into disrepute. Onyx is a gemstone that boosts self-realisation and determination, providing that extra push in manifestation and dream realisation and although it is somewhat of a contradictory stone this in no way lessens its positive effects when used by a skilled practitioner.

Peridot

Peridot or Chrysolite is one of the only stones that form in only one colour, green, the tones range from dark lime greens to olive green to lighter tones of yellowish-green but always stay within the range of 'green' with the pure lime green variety being the most sought after. Known by the Romans as the 'evening emerald' due to its resplendent light refracting properties, especially when viewed by candlelight, Peridot has also earnt the title of 'The Extreme Gem' due to the fact that (with the exception of diamond) it is the only gemstone not formed within the earth's crust but by the immense forces and molten rock that flows throughout the earth's mantle and are only brought to the surface by extreme events like volcanic eruptions and earthquakes.

Quartz (clear)

Familiar yet mysterious, this remarkable gemstone is the most abundant and commonly known gemstone on the planet. The Quartz family is vast; it is in the largest family in the mineral kingdom. Despite being so plentiful Quartz has always been highly valued and there has been a long-held belief that it is, in fact, a living being bridging the gap between animal and mineral, and one that breaths but once a century.

Red Beryl (Bixbite)

Red Beryl's extreme rarity makes it one of the world's most expensive gemstones (as high as $10.000 per carat). It is often incorrectly referred to as Red Emerald, which is incorrect as emerald is, in fact, a colour and as a gemstone Emerald actually refers to a green form of Beryl. Also known as the 'Stone of Right Time' Red Beryl is said to draw the wearer towards opportune situations and also lend a helping hand in guiding us in making the correct decision. As its name suggests Red Beryl carries a red colourisation spanning from deep yet translucent raspberry reds to lighter almost pinkish hues.

Rose Quartz

This is a 'Stone of Unconditional Love' that gets its name from its beautifully subtle shades of rose pink. It exudes a feeling of warmth and emanates compassionate energies that, through the Heart Chakra, resonates deeply with all the chakras and acts to both nourish and heal the body's energetic network as a whole. Feelings of disappointment and resentment cannot manifest in the presence of Rose Quartz and negative feeling brought into a space filled with Rose Quartz's vibrational energy will be dispelled. As a healing gemstone Rose Quartz has been used to relieve burns, stimulate and maintain a healthy heartbeat, boost fertility, treat bronchial illnesses and as an elixir has been used to treat wrinkles, boils and blisters.

Ruby

Ruby is the red variety of Corundum (other colours exist such as blue are all Sapphires) and is known as the 'King of Gems' and is one of the most valuable and sought-after gemstones on the planet, Rubies even surpassed Diamonds in ancient cultures for their magnificence, virtuosity and nobility. Ruby has an immensely influential effect on the Heart

Chakra and protects it against any unnecessary losses of energy and acts to balance the body's energy network and aura.

Sapphire

Traditionally royal blue Sapphire is a type of corundum similar to Ruby in all but colour (Rubies are in fact red corundum), however, the other colour variants are all called Sapphire. The stunning colours of the Sapphire range from royal blue to pale blue, orange, yellow, green, and pink, even purple. Sapphire is an extremely hard stone that has many practical uses beyond being fashioned into beautiful jewellery and has long been associated with royalty, prophesy and divinity in almost all religions. Sapphires have always been prized for their powerful ability to ward off evil spirits and to negate and reflect evil spells as well as supercharging the magical abilities of the user.

Selenite

Associated with the moon goddess Selene it is said that if the moon is viewed through a Selenite crystal the goddess herself can be seen. This bright crystal is a true beauty and one of the few gemstones that not only do not require charging but also boast the ability to cleanse and re-energise other crystals making Selenite highly prized by spiritualists, healers, and those adept in ancient knowledge. Known as the 'Stone of the Moon Goddess' and the 'Master Stone', Selenite's energy is in harmony with the positive end of the scale of the earth's vibrational energy field and also acts as a conduit for the tranquil energy of the moon and her many blessings.

Tourmaline

Tourmaline is a highly prized precious gemstone and is, in fact, the most colourful of all gemstones. It can be translucent or opaque and appears in hues all colours clear, white, black, blues, violets and purples, greens, browns, reds and pink, orange, yellow and even multi-coloured. The value range of Tourmaline is huge with the plainer and more common stones such as black and grey being rather modest, especially when compared to Paraiba, this neon blue/green form of Tourmaline which carries an incandescent inner glow and sells for thousands of dollars per carat, making it one of the world's most expensive gemstones.

Turquoise

Turquoise is said to be the oldest gemstone known to mankind and throughout the ages has been associated with the wisest of kings and bravest of warriors and was even used to decorate the death mask of Tutankhamun. It has been treasured for millennia as a symbol of great wisdom and ancient knowledge as well as for its protective qualities. Turquoise gets its name from the soft bluey/green hues it displays and has been used for sacred adornments, amulets and talismans that bestow luck and power for over 7000 years and it is said that Turquoise may have the ability to subtly guide or even directly lead the adept shaman towards the ultimate goal of immortality.

Chapter 8: What Influences Are The Planets On Crystals?

Sun: In our collective universe, the sun provides the collective electromagnetic energies. Corresponding to heart, freedom, leadership, joy, success, creativity, friendship, prosperity, growth, life-energy, personal-fulfilment, light, and self-confidence—the sun is also considered as the centre of the solar system and a portal to life beyond centuries. Carrying the element of Fire and the astrological sign Leo, the sun is also related to different God's and Goddess's names such as Horus, Theia, Adonis Apollo, Brigit, Vishnu-Rama-Krishna, Amaterasu, Semesh, Ilat, Ra, Bast, Hyperian, and Sekhmet. The colour of the sun is red, orange, yellow, and purple. The sun provides positive and negative electrons through the solar flare held by magnetic force. This fluid energy journey to different planets at 93 million miles per second. This energy is said to carry new, creative, and transformational power within it. Earth has its magnetic sphere called the ether, and when it reacts to the energy sent by the sun, it takes the energy efficiently and spread it to create life.

Just like earth is surrounded by ether: its electromagnetic field, we have our own electromagnetic field too. We call it the aura. The energy of our aura shines through our chakras. These expressions of ourselves when the sun reacts with the earth and the earth reacts with our body, transferring and spreading the energy of the solar flare, this magnetic expression is known as the collective consciousness. To radiate the chakras to produce the best effects in our body is to use crystals that are linked to the sun such as Citrine, Zircon, Sulfer, Heliodor, Garnet variants, and Golden Topaz. These crystals contain colours such as red, orange, yellow, blue and green. Place Citrine over your solar plexus and Heliodor over your crown chakra to boost creative thinking, personal power, attracting happiness and love, and getting rid of the people who carry a negative charge within them.

Moon: Most of us know that the moon has phases and how it revolves around the earth. Each phase of the moon carry a light that falls on the earth, but the light is less bright than the sun. It is believed that this lighter shine has negative energy embedded in its particles than of the sun during daytime, which carries positive energy. It allows the magnetic aura of the earth to be at balanced energy. Different time lengths of the earth affect the light that gets shine through the moon, also, affecting the magnetic frequency that each human body carries; hence, all the chakras.

Corresponding to clairvoyance, psychic abilities, astral travel, reincarnation, emotions, and intuition—moon also provides us with a way to enlighten ourselves through different rays. It can be achieved through meditation, yoga, and using different crystals such as Selenite, Petalite, and Moonstone that relates to the moon. It also carries the element of Water and has names related to different Gods and Goddesses such as Hecate Artemis, Sin, Mari, Khonsu, Lunah, Diana, Hathor, Atlas, and Levanah. Having the astrological sign Cancer, you can even place different crystals relating to the moon on different chakras. For instance, place Selenite on the crown chakra and Petalite on the throat chakra to balance yin and yang energies dwelling inside the body, and also, to enhance the telepathy power and intuition. Moon also have colours such as orange, yellow, green, white, and blue. The crystals under the moon contain colours such as red, orange, yellow, blue and green. These types of colours under Selenite, Petalite, and Moonstone helps the overall auric field.

Mercury: The chemical elements of mercury is very toxic, so needs to be used with caution. Named after the Roman God, it is known to provide affinities to the mental faculties such as thoughts, creative writing, reasoning, communication, and other elements related to air. Also, corresponding to wisdom, science, cleverness—it has an astrological sign of Virgo and Gemini. Virgo is associated with analytical abilities, understanding one's experiences, and the ability to develop intuition, while Gemini is associated with the rational mind, collecting information, clearing thoughts, and pursuing knowledge.

Crystals relating to mercury are Fire Agate and Blue Lace Agate. It also carries the names of God and Goddess such as Metis, Woden, Anubis, Maat, Hermes, Athena, and Thoth. The colour that mercury represents is blue, yellow, pink, purple mixed, blue, and grey. Place the Fire Agate crystal over the base or root chakra and place the Blue Lace Agate over the throat or third chakra to feel the flow of kinaesthetic energy to bring a sense of equilibrium in the body. This combination also helps in to ease with anger and frustration.

Venus: The second planet from the sun, Venus is named after the Roman goddess. This planet is high in temperature, twice the solar radiation that emits out from the earth. Pressure dense atmosphere containing sulfuric acid, Venus corresponds to pleasure, love, luxury, beauty, and the arts. Having the elements of Earth and Water, Venus is also ninety-five times greater than the earth. Accompanied by the tarot of The Empress, Venus also represents different crystals such as Amazonite, Rose Quartz, and Emerald.

A thick cloud covers around the area of Venus, once every four-day rotating much faster than the planet. Also, having mountains and metal, just like earth, Venus can be seen from the naked eye from the Earth, including night and day.

Venus also is known by the name of the Gods and Goddesses such as Pan, Inanna, Venus, Eros, Hathor, Ishtar, Oceanus, and Aphrodite. Venus represents the colour white, yellow, light blue, and light green. Place Rose quartz over your heart chakra and Amazonite over the throat to activate self-love, empathy, and forgiveness along with enhanced communication skills and balancing the masculine and feminine energies.

Mars: The iron oxide appearing on the surface of mars concludes its other name as the red planet. Having its name from the Roman god of war, Mars is half the size comparing to earth. Two moons orbit around the planet of mars. Accompanied by the element Fire, it also corresponds to the crystals such as Ruby, Red Jasper, and Garnet. Mars is also the planet that is to be inhibited by humans soon. The planet can also be seen through the earth without the requirement of the telescope.

Mars also represents the astrological signs such as Scorpio and Aries. The possibility of life can be traced there because deep down there is an ocean too, buried deep comparable to the height of Mount Everest. Mars is also referred with Gods and Goddesses name such as Diana, Tyr, Morrigan, Heracles, Anath, Horus, Aries, and Brigit. Garnet helps in cleaning all the chakras while placing ruby over the heart chakra and Red Jasper over base or root chakra, it sets the foundation for spiritual and physical energy of the body, expanding the expression of love.

Jupiter: The biggest planet in our solar system, Jupiter is named after the mythological king of gods. Having lots of moon and different rocky bands revolving around it, Jupiter also corresponds to inspiration, wisdom, teacher, honour, justice, and generosity. In regards to the astrology, Jupiter represents the principle of assimilation and expansion. It tells us to learn and go beyond our limits. Telling us to participate in our belief system, while chasing our goals and spiritual quest, Jupiter also carries the element of Fire and Air.

The relating crystals such as Azurite, Lapiz Lazuli, and White Topaz, Jupiter also has Sagittarius as an astrological sign. The positive qualities that Jupiter include are love, faith, cheerfulness, and trust. Jupiter also represents the colour such as green, yellow, brown, purple, and white. Place Lapiz Lazuli over the third eye, Azurite over the crown chakra to experience great psychic gift as well as getting rid of any blockage in other chakras. Jupiter also has other names of Gods and Goddesses such as Juno, Zeus, Themis, Thor, Isia, Hera, and Marduk.

Saturn: It is the kind of planet which is known for gambling, obstinacy, and chronic diseases. It also regulates death and ageing, hunters and thieves, foreign travel, and yoga practice. While this planet is not good for people, but if it is placed rightly then it provides great balance in different virtues such as longevity, compassion, charity, and meditative insight. Also, corresponding to limitations, knowledge, institutions, boundaries, discipline, and obstacle, the element it carries is Earth. Having the astrological sign Capricorn, Saturn, if powerful, can allow the person to be an affectionate mate and can also provide longevity. If not, if the Saturn is weak, then the person can become vulnerable, having headaches and other nervous system problems.

Known by God's and Goddess's such as Rhea, Green Man, Hecate, Saturn, Hera, Cronus, Kali, Demeter, and Nephthys— Saturn spreads its cosmic energy through Indicolite, Amethyst, Blue Spinel, Blue Sapphires, Lodestone, Jet, Hematite, and Onyx. Saturn also represents the colour such as black, ashy, white, pale and dark colours. Place Blue Spinel over throat chakra and Hematite over root chakra to stay grounded, to convert negative energy into positive energy, and to enable excellent non-judgemental communication.

Uranus: Found in 1781, Uranus brings sudden changes that are both interpersonal and collective, appearing out of nowhere. Corresponding to sufficiency, untapped potential, independence, originality, and freedom, it also carries the element of Air. The sudden changes that bring a very high energy intensity, it will require time to settle, but it also offers new insights and a higher level of awareness in an individual's life. Uranus challenges the person to take immediate measure to initiate order in his/ her life to set their values and perspective.

Having the astrological sign Aquarius, Uranus is known by the name of Gods and Goddesses such as Pan, Isis, and Zeus. The electromagnetic charge that this planet carries, it can effectively wreck the nervous system, causing anxiety and insomnia. Uranus ignites the process of clairvoyance in an individual, allowing them to see things as they are so that they can synthesize their thoughts, ideas, and actions into a flexible structure. Kyanite and Amethyst can also help in this. Other crystals related to Uranus are Diamond and Quartz. Place Diamond at the crown chakra to bring the balance of the energy and use Quartz to align all the chakras through harmony. The colours that this planet represents are the different colours of the green spectrum.

Neptune: Named after the Roman gods of the seas, this planet is associated with intuition, dreams, extra-terrestrial dimensions, arts, and unconditional love. It also tries to explore what lay beneath the surface of consciousness, expands the mystical experiences along with understanding the transcendental reality. To attune with Neptune's energy, crystals such as Tanzanite, Aquamarine, and Lapiz Lazuli can be used. It also corresponds to personal insights, divinity, emotions, endurance, and inspiration. Known by the Gods and Goddesses such as Ishtar and Neptune, its astrological sign is Pisces.

Its experiences also include the need for releasing emotions, the karmic issues from this life or previous life. Other experience can relate to the inability to suffer the burdens of this physical world, but it also offers the opportunity to become something more, a higher human being, taking actions and expanding awareness. Other crystals to soak in the energy of Neptune are Jade and Sapphire. Place the Sapphire into the third eye and Jade over the heart chakra to experience mental clarity and harmony to bring emotional and physical balance. The colour that Neptune represents is deep blue and light blue.

Pluto: This planet can influence money, sex, and power. Also, corresponding to transformation, renewal, spirituality, rebirth, and self-knowledge, it carries the element of Fire. To get attuned to the energy of Pluto, use Obsidian, Topaz, Smoky Quartz, and Ruby. Pluto is also known by the names of Gods and Goddesses such as Persephone, Pluto, and Osiris. The colour represents are dark green, speckled black, dark blue, and Black. Place Obsidian over the root chakra and Ruby over the heart chakra to increase self-control and the flow of loving emotions to express love. This also helps with stress and anxiety.

Chapter 9: Stop Ringing In The Ears - Use Remedies For Tinnitus To Stop The Awful Noise

When you experience the ill effects of ear ringing tinnitus, you will realize how terrible it can turn into. With the commotion in your ears gradually making you insane as it ends up more intense and progressively visit.

It can and makes you sick with the worry of attempting to live with it. When you begin to think there is nothing you can do about it and the humming ears will deteriorate this will make frantic for solutions for tinnitus.

There are different reasons for these commotions and ringing in the ear. Vast numbers of them can be treated with a prescription. In any case, if it is identified with hearing misfortune or introduction to the noisy commotion, at that point prescription won't help, this is because there is physical harm to the ears.

If you have been recommended prescription or medications you know, they send in a cabinet as they don't do anything to help.

There are essential medicines for tinnitus that work by treating the triggers and reasons for these commotions and are demonstrated to work. A few reasons for tinnitus can be treated with a prescription, for example, ear contaminations, yet the sort that a great many people experience the ill effects of medicine can't manage, and this is the sort brought about by hearing misfortune or boisterous clamor.

As it turns out to be more regrettable, the commotion can cause you restless evenings and anticipate you hearing what individuals are stating to you. It can even power you to leave your place of employment.

Introduction to uproarious commotion leaves your hearing in danger of permanent harm. If you hear ringing in your ears after being presented to boisterous clamor, it is essential to find a way to stop tinnitus. Finding a way to stay away from the noisy commotion and utilizing earplugs around uproarious clamors will avert tinnitus ending up more terrible, yet it won't stop it.

Homeopathic cures are demonstrated to work, by treating the causes, regardless of whether you have suffered from the loathsome ringing of the ears for a considerable length of time.

If you are searching for solutions for tinnitus utilize homeopathic solutions for additional help from the ringing in your ears and recover your life.

Treat Angular Cheilitis Using Remedies Produced From Plants

Rakish cheilitis is a condition which influences the mouth territory that is likewise called stomatitis, perleche, and here and there, just 'cheilitis.' This horrifying condition often shows as coarse, red zones around the mouth and parallel injuries on either side of the mouth territory where the upper and lower lips associate. It's brought about by an over developing of oral germs and may be joined by auxiliary contagious contamination.

It is imperative to ultimately get a handle on what rakish cheilitis is and what causes it all together that it tends to be dealt with as needs are. Perleche isn't connected to the infection that prompts mouth blisters, and fever rankles and regarding it as though it can cause significantly more inconvenience. It is prudent to visit a doctor if you get any unexplained injuries and distress around the mouth zone and, if it is cheilitis, you will most likely be given cortisone or some antifungal treatment to help fix it. Cortisone utilized to treat precise cheilitis often stirs very well in clearing up the condition, yet it's risky. A few people accept that it diminishes the skin and that the epidermis encompassing the mouth region is never the equivalent after utilizing it. It's likewise felt that cortisone stimulates fat addition when taken orally yet it's only from time to time endorsed in tablet structure to treat stomatitis aside from if there's a great deal of discharge and horrible draining and topical medicine may be confusing and challenging to utilize.

Even though manufactured prescriptions carry out the responsibility for the time being, they are not the ideal approach to treat precise cheilitis in the long haul. That is the place organic cures gotten from plants come in. Numerous natural cures can be securely used in the long haul and with no unfavorable impacts. Plant-inferred arrangements are also more pleasant to work with and might be a piece of safeguard measures notwithstanding treatment for perleche.

Australian tea tree and aloe vera are two plants much of the time utilized in the treating stomatitis and are available in cream, gel, ointment, and lip-demulcent structure. Tea tree is besides widely accessible as oil and even a mouth wash which functions admirably to annihilate the microbes in the mouth as well as to wipe out the yeast contamination that much of the time happens with cheilitis. Tea tree is a solid disinfectant, hostile to the bacterial and calming operator which is utilized to fix an assortment of infirmities, not simply precise stomatitis. Nectar is likewise sterile, albeit made by honey bees, is one increasingly common and plant-determined item that can be utilized to address the condition topically. Cocoa margarine things produced using the fat of the cocoa bean are exceptionally mitigating when connected to influenced spots as cream or lip emollient. It's additionally conceivable to utilize a blend produced using squashed garlic and olive leaves, and citrus and tea tree oils, to specify only a couple.

People who wear dentures often experience the ill effects of perleche as microbes can develop on the dentures and get caught in the hole in the middle of severely fitting dentures and the gums. Like this a couple of drops of tea tree oil in the water used to absorb the dentures is an approach to in a roundabout way treat rakish cheilitis and to shield microscopic organisms from developing on your dentures.

Use Remedy For Beard Patches

Everybody likes to search tremendous and for that person do a wide range of endeavors. When people don't look great, then they become less sure of themselves? There are countless items which guarantee to make people increasingly excellent. Such a significant number of people utilize such things and attempt to make themselves progressively attractive. There are such a large number of organizations which are making plenty of benefits by offering such items to people at present. Why it is so significant for people to look fabulous?

Indeed, there are numerous purposes for this. In the first place, people feel upbeat from inside when they look great. Second, when people look great, then they regularly get compliments from a few people, and this lifts their fearlessness. Third, great looks help people in simply blending with others. Numerous people don't think that its simple at all to begin a discussion with other people as a result of how they look. Practically all people like to deal with their appearance. Numerous people feel that solitary ladies should focus on their appearance; however, it isn't the situation.

Men regularly utilize a few items which help them in looking attractive. There is plenty of men who like to deal with their appearance. The present period is a time of metrosexual men who want to spoil themselves. Men frequently prefer to develop their facial hair as they look hot in it. There may be numerous people who don't care to build their whiskers in light of facial hair patches. Any individual who is encountering the issue of whiskers patches should realize that this issue can be dealt with. The vast majority believe that it can't be dealt with and they continue bearing it.

It is additionally conceivable that a few people don't have a clue about what they are experiencing such fixes. However, they are. When anybody needs to comprehend what this condition is called, then we might want to refer to the name of alopecia barbae. The issue of alopecia barbae isn't new, and from old ages, countless men experience this issue. At the point when people experience the ill effects of any medical problem, then they regularly visit their primary care physician. One ought to consistently attempt to discover the arrangement of a problem. There may be numerous explanations behind which people are not ready to find an answer to this issue.

Any individual who needs to think about the alopecia barbae treatment needs to sign on to the web. One will go over an enormous number of websites which offer data about the cures of this issue. In any case, people should depend on rumored sites.

One can, without much of a stretch, discover the alopecia barbae treatment with the assistance of the web. Presently days, the internet is utilized by people for countless reasons. At whatever point, people need to get some data about anything; then they use the web.

Angular Cheilitis Symptoms and Some Useful Remedies

When you appear to have dry split skin at the edges of your mouth, especially during the virus winter months, you have rakish cheilitis symptoms. There might be profound parts or splits into one of the two sides of the mouth, and they may move toward becoming excited even to the point of draining and maybe getting to be contaminated.

If the condition is left untreated, it might end up contaminated by an organism called Candida albicans or thrush. Studies have demonstrated the issue might be connected to nutrient or wholesome lacks sometimes, especially riboflavin (nutrient B2), just as Zinc inadequacy and iron insufficiency weakness. Now and again older individuals have known to show rakish cheilitis symptoms because of their dentures not fitting effectively, or they might miss teeth through and through, and making them over close their mouth or shut it on one side more so than the other.

For the most part, when precise cheilitis symptoms emerge in colder months, for example, in wintertime, they might be analyzed as having cheilitis; however, it is only a cut off an instance of dried out lips. Kids particularly may lick their mouths, trying to dampen them and make a considerably more severe issue for themselves. The makes keep running from attack from microscopic organisms parasitic diseases.

Treatment or cures incorporate the utilization of a topical disinfectant cream which must be connected to the zone of soreness for a few days. When there is contamination included, the individual influenced must utilize some over the counter antifungal cream, and if the condition continues, a specialist ought to be looked for counsel. The precise cheilitis symptoms will, by and large, die down without anyone else inside a couple of days if the region is kept clean and cream is connected.

In some instances including severely dry and broke skin about the mouth territory, a malabsorption disorder might be to be faulted, making precise cheilitis symptoms. Giving nutrient B-12 shots may demonstrate helpfully, or even whole B complex shots might be advised. This will be resolved by the seriousness of the signs and how well the tissue reacts to the utilization of the disinfectant or antifungal cream at first connected.

A lack of a significant number of B nutrients can be the reason for rakish cheilitis symptoms. These incorporate niacin (B3), pyridoxine (B6), riboflavin (B2), and cyanocobalamin (B12). Acidic corrosive can fuel the condition, and drinking squeezed an orange, or lemonade may make the mouth become dryer and splitting to increment. Guidance from a specialist is exceptionally prescribed to discount contamination and parasitic illnesses.

Avoiding Female Balding Naturally - Don't Use Remedies Created For Men!

Numerous individuals consider thinning up top and balding as being just a male issue, yet that isn't the situation by any stretch of the imagination.

It is evaluated that sooner or later in their lives, around 66% of ladies will experience the ill effects of male pattern baldness.

And keeping in mind that it is moderately uncommon for ladies to turn out to be bare, it is none the less a significant issue for the ladies concerned.

Female going bald, which as a rule brings about diminishing of the hair everywhere throughout the scalp, has various causes, some of which are hormonal.

Notwithstanding the reason most ladies who experience the ill effects of this female example hair loss, as it is known, naturally feel delicate about the condition, and this can build their feelings of anxiety.

These, expanded feelings of anxiety at that point proceeds with the cycle and... all things considered, you needn't bother with me to work the end.

Interestingly, there are presently options accessible, which will take care of the issue. Also, the far superior news is that there are a few items, which contain just regular organic fixings to accomplish a compelling arrangement.

Whereas in the past ladies who were enduring with male pattern baldness issues needed to depend on utilizing hair reestablishing items intended for men, with every one of the problems that came about because of doing as such, things are currently evolving.

Not exclusively are their items, yet they are structured explicitly for the requirements of the female body!

The critical fixings in these items contrast just because people have altogether different prerequisites, and that has had a massive effect on the outcomes ladies are currently encountering in hair re-development.

With a usual mix of horsetail together with nutrients and minerals, for example, Zinc, Biotin, and Magnesium, the containers can rapidly and viably lessen female thinning up top.

Headache Home Remedies That Can Help

Headache is an ailment that includes synthetic concoctions in the body. These synthetic compounds, for example, serotonin, when present in abnormal states, causes blood levels to choke. The abrupt drop in levels of these synthetics causes the veins to all of a sudden to widen and develop to come about to a headache. Albeit much is thought about problems, specialists still don't have the foggiest idea of how to fix it. This makes it extremely confused to manage. What most specialists and headache patients do is to utilize cures in the types of prescriptions and treatments that help people arrangement and adapt up to a headache, and it's going with manifestations.

The most widely recognized type of managing headaches incorporates drugs, for example, analgesics, non-steroid mitigating medications. These give moment help. There are cases wherein it causes more agony than alleviation; subsequently, a few people pick different types of cures.

A few types of home treatment and the physical procedure can be considered as elective home solutions for headaches. One is needle therapy. This method includes embeddings needles into determined focuses to impact the equalization of the body. The point of this strategy is to animate the arrival of endorphins, change the thoughtful and autonomic sensory systems, and to invigorate and improve blood dissemination. Needle therapy has demonstrated to be viable for helping people manage torment and wounds just as forestalling cerebral pains, muscle stresses, and fits. Another is biofeedback. Biofeedback enables an individual to deliberately change and control the body's vital capacities that are regularly oblivious. After much training, processes, for example, breathing and the pulse can be controlled with the psyche. Different structures incorporate message treatment and hydrotherapy, outer utilization of water in various fabrics to a piece of the human body. It tends to be finished utilizing materials found at home, for example, hot and ice water. These materials help in blood dissemination. These elective home cures manage the physical condition of the individual.

Another elective cure considered by bounty is taking in herbs. These cures, for the most part, manage the admission of the individual enduring headaches. Here and there, it fills in as enhancements to people to diminish the side effects they feel and to further reduce the odds of problems happening what's to come. One such herb is cayenne. It contains capsaicin which is accepted to obstruct a concoction that is engaged with agony transmission in the nerves. A few examinations have demonstrated that patients who take in cayenne encountered a noteworthy reduction in the force of torment during their headaches. Ginger, a herb generally found in the kitchen, decreases pain due to its mitigating properties. It has likewise been seen that ginger declines the propensity of blood platelets to cluster together, lessening the head torment present in headaches.

These home cures or medicines can be viable with headaches. In any case, most specialists and authority must be counseled when considering these elective cures. It is always conceivable that these elective cures, rather than helping an individual arrangement with headache, can further disturb the circumstance by methods for hypersensitivities and included cerebral pains, and so on.

Home Remedies For Acne On Face

As skin break out can be considered as the skin rashes with no specific purpose for, it can not be taken a gander at like the genuine medical problem. In any case, once in a while, it came about into scratches. The skin breaks out affected mostly at the territories of face, neck, back, chest, and shoulders. One of the upsetting affected regions of Acne is the face, which results in a bothered condition from where individuals ended up unsociable.

As there is no specific explanation for the event of skin inflammation other than hormonal lopsidedness, the cure of this skin issue includes, for the most part, the regular treatment. According to a drug, one can take anti-infection. There are some home remedies present for restoring this skin issue. To give some examples, they are:

After Cooking oatmeal, one needs to apply this cooked oatmeal on the face for fifteen minutes.

To diminish the skin inflammation, one needs to clean up with whiten of annoy and rosemary.

Applying adequate measure of lemon squeeze and rose water with a cotton ball additionally diminishes skin break out issue. In the wake of using this blend, it should be left for 30 minutes and after that wash off. This cure should be rehashed for 15-20 days.

Snagging the skin inflammation with garlic cloves additionally diminishes skin break out. This cure needs to apply a few times each day.

The mixture of avocado glue and water is another home solution for skin inflammation issue.

'Bedouin drugs' is additionally another home cure that includes few stages to cure the skin inflammation issue. These means are: Having a medium ground radish with every dinner and drinking of 2 cups of rosemary tea and alcohol of 3 glasses of water with crushed lemon and nectar.

The mixture of 1 tablespoon of dried or new yeast and two tablespoons of lemon squeeze likewise lessens skin inflammation issue. The blend should be connected on the face, and one needs to hold up until it gets hard. After that, the cover should be stripped off with warm water.

To keep away from and confine the development of skin break out on the face, one needs to clear the surface all the time with an absorbed cotton ball either lemon juice or apple juice vinegar.

I am mixing of 2-3 tea packs to some basil and after that after cooked in bubbling water for 10-20 minutes. This blend should be connected on the skin inflammation with a cotton ball.

The water which is immersed with lettuce leaves is qualified to apply on the skin inflammation.

Ground narrows leaves alongside whitening in the water likewise helps in diminishing skin break out on the face.

Boiled water with included apple juice vinegar additionally accommodating in lessening the skin break out issue. The vapor of this blend should have been taken.

One straightforward solution for this issue is to abstain from contacting the affected region.

I am applying of toothpaste just before hitting the sack likewise a helpful solution for skin break out.

A glue of new fenugreek leaves over the face likewise decreases the issue.

A paste of neem leaves alongside turmeric is an ayurvedic however home solution for skin inflammation on the face.

Explanations behind Surge in Natural Remedies

In late decades, usual remedies and cures have seen a strong resurgence in fame. It might appear to be strange that when therapeutic innovation is expanding at such a fast rate, that individuals would turn out to be progressively keen on exploring and utilizing remedies that have been around for hundreds and, sometimes, a great many years. It is, in any case, the consequence of these very advances in medicinal science and research that are demonstrating that numerous common remedies are totally protected as well as amazingly powerful. There are various reasons why attempting a characteristic cure can be a decent alternative rather than quickly looking for pharmacological help.

Conclusion

Nature has blessed you with its helping hand in the form of crystals. You can make the most of your life by sprinkling this magic into different aspects of it. You have been provided here with the necessary essentials for you to start your crystal healing journey. Make most of what you have learned in this book by choosing the perfect crystals for yourself, and incorporate different crystal energies into different tasks to achieve optimal results. A complete directory has been provided to you in order to offer you guidance at every step of the initial journey. With these fundamentals you now have the ability to purchase the perfect crystal fitting your needs.

It is highly important that you stick to the purchasing and selection guidelines provided here in order to build a strong relationship with your first crystal. The journey that you will embark upon is truly a spiritual one.

Finally, with the different charging and activation techniques explained to you here, you now have the power to use a single crystal for multiple benefits. Make sure you manage the crystal in the best way possible. Do not forget to clean your crystal in order to maintain its positive healing powers.

Your life is about to change for good. Your new crystal will surely revolutionize your entire world in the best way possible, provided you use it in accordance to this guidance. Now you can finally begin an entirely new life and an entirely different you.